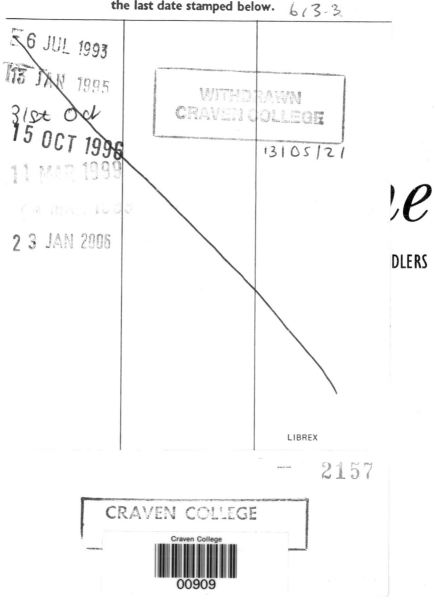

*e*

DLERS

# Hygiene

## A COMPLETE COURSE FOR FOOD HANDLERS

*Hazelwood & McLean*

Hodder & Stoughton

LONDON SYDNEY AUCKLAND TORONTO

The author and publishers would like to thank the following organisations for permission to reproduce copyright material: The Hotel Catering and Institutional Management Association for the diagram on p. 18 and the Dept. Health and MAFF for the 'Ten Golden Rules' on p. 115. The 'Main reasons for food poisoning' which appears on pp. 33 and 34 are attributed to Dr D Roberts, Food Hygiene Laboratory, Central Public Health Laboratory, Colindale and was originally produced for the Institution of Environmental Health Officers 'Food Hygiene Handbook'.

British Library Cataloguing in Publication Data

Hazelwood, David
   Hygiene: a complete course for food handlers.
   I. Title
   363.1907

   ISBN 0–340–56165–3

First published 1991

Typeset by Wearside Tradespools, Boldon, Tyne and Wear.
Printed in Great Britain for the educational publishing division of Hodder & Stoughton Ltd, Mill Road, Dunton Green, Sevenoaks, Kent by St Edmundsbury Press Ltd.

# CONTENTS

# INTRODUCTION

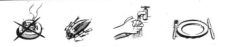

Everyone who is employed in the food industry today requires approved training in basic food hygiene in order to comply with The Food Safety Act 1990.

This pack is designed to allow you to work on your own and at your own pace. There is no pressure on you to have work completed by a certain date.

Don't think that you know nothing about food hygiene – a lot of it is common sense and you will be surprised just how much you already know. Don't worry if you haven't done exams for a number of years because food hygiene examinations are just like filling in questionnaires in a magazine. All you usually have to do is tick boxes or circle numbers to answer the questions.

## How to use this training package

The package is divided into fifteen sections, each one dealing with a particular aspect of food hygiene, and you can complete these sections in any order you choose. Before starting the package you should glance through it to get acquainted with the layout and familiarise yourself with each section. Do not try and complete too many sections at one time. (Two sections in any one learning period is sufficient.) You still need time between each section to think about and understand the knowledge you have gained.

At the end of each section there is a short revision test for you to complete and assess the knowledge you have gained. (Some of these tests require short written answers, but this is to expand your understanding of the subject – most final examination questions can be answered with a tick or a circle.) Read through the relevant section again after you have answered the questions and then, *and only then*, check your answer with the answers in the back of the package.

Whilst you are at work, relate the sections you have covered to your working environment and discuss points, including those about which you are unsure, with fellow students, colleagues and supervisors. Involve them in the course: the reason you are doing this course is to improve and maintain food hygiene standards in order to prevent the increasing incidences of food poisoning which occur annually.

Once you have completed all the sections in the package – and gone over those sections you were not too sure about – there is an ENDTEST to complete. This is, if you like, a mock examination. Allow yourself a maximum of forty minutes to complete the ENDTEST under examination conditions – no TV, stereos or interruptions.

# How colleges and learning centres can use this package for full time, part time, open-learning and company employed students

Food hygiene is an integrated part of all food handlers' tuition, but until now may not have been validated by a nationally recognised examination.

This training package is suitable for City & Guilds, BTEC Catering, Leisure & Hospitality, Nursery Nurses and Caring courses – in fact every course where the participant is likely to handle food.

The Food Safety Act requires that *all* food handlers receive training in this essential area up to approved examination standards.

This package – *HYGIENE: A COMPLETE COURSE FOR FOOD HANDLERS* – can be used by all students without formal classroom sessions, so allowing them to complete the course at their own pace without using expensive human, time and accommodation resources.

Full time and part time students can purchase the package, as essential reading, to complete in their own time. Structured 'think–ins' can be built into existing practical learning sessions to help consolidate the knowledge gained.

Open-learning students can purchase the package to complete, as for other students. Again, formal 'think-in' sessions can be arranged, a telephone 'chat-line' arranged for tutorial purposes, or tutorial sessions held on clients premises where companies are using the package to train staff in-house (subject to the relevant fees for this service being met in addition to the cost of this package).

# LEARNING TARGET

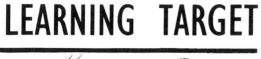

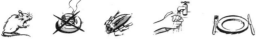

After completing this training package you will:

◆ Know the standards of personal hygiene required of food handlers

◆ Know the causes of food poisoning

◆ Know how to prevent food poisoning

◆ Know how to dispose of waste food safely, without contributing to cross – contamination

◆ Know how to use refrigerators and freezers to avoid cross – contamination and store food safely

◆ Know and be able to operate the safe stock rotation of food stuffs

◆ Know the common pests found in food premises and how to control them

◆ Know and be able to operate the safe and hygienic cleaning procedures

◆ Know how food legislation affects you and operate within the guidelines which are laid down

# SECTION ONE

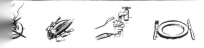

# Terminology

As you work your way through this training package you will come across some technical terms which are used to describe certain aspects of food hygiene.

The terms used are specific to food hygiene, just as the terms 'crank shaft', 'piston', 'differential' or 'carburettor' would be necessary if you were learning about the workings of the engine of a car. They are not intended to make the subject appear difficult. Spend as long as is necessary learning these terms before going any further with your studies.

## Terms used throughout food hygiene training package

**Bacterium (bacteria pl.)**   A living organism which is invisible to the naked eye, some forms of which can cause food poisoning if allowed to multiply and grow without control. (Often called a 'bug' or 'germ'.)

**Detergent**   A chemical which is used to help remove dirt, grease and debris from a surface before disinfection.

**Disinfectant**   A chemical which reduces harmful bacteria to a safe level.

**Carrier**   A person who harbours or may pass on harmful bacteria without showing signs of illness themselves.

**Contamination**   The presence of any objectionable matter in food – either bacteria, metal, poison or anything which makes the food unsuitable for people to eat.

**Cross – contamination**   A process when the bacteria from one area are moved, usually by a food handler, to another area and so infect foods or surfaces etc. in an otherwise clean area. (*Most dangerous instances of CROSS – CONTAMINATION occur when a food handler moves from handling raw meats to cooked foods without washing their hands!*)

**Food handler**   Anyone who is employed in the production, preparation, processing, packaging, storage, transport, distribution and sale of food.

**Food poisoning**   A very unpleasant illness which can last for a number of days and is caused by eating contaminated foodstuffs.

**High risk foods**   Foods which have a high protein content and readily support bacterial growth and will not be cooked again before eating.

**Onset period**   The length of time between eating infected food and the first signs of illness.

**Spoilage**   A process in food which makes the food unsuitable for human consumption through incorrect or prolonged storage.

**Sanitiser**   A combination detergent and disinfectant.

**Spoilage bacteria**   Bacteria which cause food to be spoiled and so unfit for human consumption, but do not necessarily cause food poisoning.

**Spores**   A resistant resting-phase of bacteria which protects them against extremes of temperature.

*Now complete the following questions at your own pace. When you have completed the questions, check your answers by reading through Section 1 again. Mark your answers using the answer grid on page 3*

**Which food hygiene terms do the following descriptions refer to?**

1 _____

Living organisms which are invisible to the naked eye, some forms of which can cause food poisoning if allowed to multiply and grow without control. (Often called 'bugs' or 'germs').

2 _____

A chemical which is used to help remove dirt, grease and debris from a surface before disinfection.

3 _____

A chemical which reduces harmful bacteria to a safe level.

4 _____

The presence of any objectionable matter in food – either bacteria, metal, poison or anything which makes the food unsuitable for people to eat.

5 _____ _____

A process when the bacteria from one area are moved, usually by a food handler, to another area and so infect foods or surfaces etc. in an otherwise clean area.
(*Most dangerous instance occurs when food handlers move from handling raw meats to cooked foods without washing their hands!*)

6 ____ _____

Anyone who is employed in the production, preparation, processing, packaging, storage, transport, distribution and sale of food.

7 ____ _____

A very unpleasant illness which can last for a number of days and is caused by eating contaminated foodstuffs.

8 ____ ____ _____

Foods which have a high protein content and readily support bacterial growth and which will not be cooked again before eating.

9 _____

A combination detergent and disinfectant.

# SECTION TWO

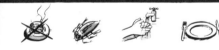

# *What is food hygiene?*

To most people the word hygiene means *cleanliness*. If something looks clean then they think that it must also be hygienic. As someone employed in the food handling industry you must do everything in your power to make certain that the food you handle is 100% hygienic and safe to eat without causing food poisoning.

The true definition of food hygiene is:

◆ The destruction of all and any harmful bacteria in the food by thorough cooking or other processes

◆ The protection of the food from contamination, including harmful bacteria, foreign bodies and poisons

◆ The prevention of the multiplication of harmful bacteria to the degree where illness of the consumer occurs or the prevention of premature spoilage of the food itself

It is essential that good hygiene practices within the food premises are carried out as a matter of course by *all* staff if food which is truly hygienic is to be sold.

This Basic Food Hygiene training package has been designed specially to allow you to learn these practices and so work safely and in an hygienic manner, although knowing the practices is not enough. You must put what you have learnt into use and make sure that you follow the practices *at all times*.

Once you thoroughly understand the need for hygiene practices then it is very unlikely that you will work in anything other than a hygienic manner. Poor hygiene practices are usually the result of ignorance and carelessness and can have very serious consequences both for yourself and your employers.

# The costs of poor hygiene practices

Closure of the business

Loss of your job

Heavy fines and legal costs and possible imprisonment

Loss of your reputation

Payment of compensation to food poisoning victims

Food poisoning outbreaks and even death

Contaminated food and complaints from customers and staff

◆ Food waste due to spoilage

Staff with a poor morale and therefore lacking pride in their work which means a high staff turnover and less money for wages, bonus payments etc.

It is not only your employer who could be prosecuted if a food poisoning outbreak occurs. If you were found to be responsible then you too could be prosecuted and you would find it very difficult to get another job in the food industry!

# Benefits of good hygiene practices

A good personal and business reputation

Increased yields from foodstuffs which results in greater profitability and higher wage levels

A high staff morale which results in a happier, safer working environment

Satisfied customers

Good working conditions with lower staff turnover

Complying with the law and a happy and satisfied Public Protection Department. (Looking over your shoulder for the 'Public health man' can be very stressful.)

Personal and job satisfaction

Would you rather work in premises which have poor standards of hygiene or those which have high standards?

*Now complete the following questions at your own pace. When you have completed the questions, check your answers by reading through Section 2 again. Mark your answers using the answer grid at the end of package*

**I**   Which statement would best describe *'good food hygiene'*?

   *a*   keeping all food surfaces clean
   *b*   protection of food from contamination
   *c*   washing your hands after every activity
   *d*   not allowing pests in the food area

**2**   Fill in the missing words in the following sentences to complete the definitions of *'food hygiene'*.

Spoilage    Poisons     Bacteria
Cooking     Harmful     Contamination
Bacteria    Illness     Multiplication

   *a*   the *destruction* of all and any _____ bacteria in the food by thorough _____ or other process.

   *b*   the *protection* of the food from _____ including harmful _____, foreign bodies and _____.

   *c*   the *prevention* of the _____ of existing _____ to the degree where _____ of the consumer occurs or the prevention of premature _____ of the food itself.

# SECTION THREE

# Personal hygiene

Whenever there is a case of food poisoning there is *always* one cause. . . . HUMAN.

Food poisoning does not 'just happen', it is caused, and it is *always* caused by someone not following good hygiene practices. It is therefore essential that you follow a strict routine of *personal hygiene* so that good hygiene practices can occur. Food poisoning organisms are present, at one time or another, on everyone, no matter how careful they are over their personal hygiene. If you are employed in the food industry you have both a *legal* and *moral* obligation to make sure that the food you handle is not contaminated by your lack of personal hygiene.

## Areas of personal hygiene

The areas of personal hygiene you must be most careful about are:

Hands and skin

Cuts, boils, septic spots, grazes etc.

Hair

Ear, nose and mouth

Smoking

Wearing jewellery, perfume and aftershave

Protective clothing

◆ General health care and reporting of illness

◆ Hygiene education

## *HANDS AND SKIN*

If you are working with food, your hands must come into contact with the food. It is therefore essential that your hands are as hygienic as possible *at all times*. It is not sufficient simply to wash your hands before you begin work. Throughout your working day your hands will be in contact with surfaces, foods and substances which carry harmful bacteria or germs and there is a very great risk of *cross–contamination* leading to outbreaks of food poisoning.

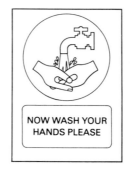

NOW WASH YOUR
HANDS PLEASE

Your hands must be washed every time you change activities during your working day, especially when you move from preparing or handling raw meats and foods to preparing or handling cooked meats and foods.

Hands should be washed (in the wash hand basin provided specifically for that purpose) with a bactericidal soap, nails scrubbed with the nail brush provided and dried thoroughly . . .

◆ After using the w.c.

◆ In between handling raw and cooked foods

◆ After combing your hair

◆ On entering the food preparation area and before using equipment or handling any food

◆ After eating, smoking or blowing your nose

◆ After handling refuse or waste food

You should be most particular about wearing clean underclothes and showering or bathing regularly to make sure that you do not harbour harmful bacteria on your skin and so suffer the embarrassment of body odour (B.O.).

Fingernails should be kept trimmed very short as long nails harbour many harmful bacteria. Nail varnish should not be worn by food handlers as particles can become dislodged and cause contamination and spoilage of food. Allowing your fingers to come into contact with your mouth in any way, whilst handling food, must be stopped. The most common 'crime' which food handlers commit is to lick their fingers before separating sheets of greaseproof paper, paper bags etc.

## CUTS, BOILS, SEPTIC SPOTS, GRAZES etc.

Any breakage of skin is an *ideal* place for bacteria to multiply. All skin breakages must be covered with a waterproof, coloured dressing to protect against cross-contamination.

*Why coloured?* Food handlers must wear coloured waterproof dressings so that, if they become dislodged and fall into foodstuffs during preparation, they can be identified quickly and easily and the food disposed of.

## HAIR

Hair is a particularly 'unclean' aspect of your personal hygiene. Your hair is constantly falling out and contains dandruff; both find their way into food and cause contamination. Regular shampooing of hair is necessary by food handlers as the scalp often contains harmful bacteria. *All* food handlers must wear suitable head gear so that their hair is completely covered.

This also includes beards, which must be covered by a suitable face mask or beard net.

Your hair should not be combed whilst you are wearing protective clothing as stray hair and dandruff can end up on the clothes and be transferred into the food.

## EAR, NOSE AND MOUTH

One type of bacteria we shall be discussing later in the training package is *Staphylococcus* which is found in the nose and mouth of 40–45% of adults.

    *Staphylococci* (pl) contribute to many cases of food poisoning and are spread very easily when you sneeze, cough or even whistle whilst in the food areas. If you are suffering from a cold you must not be allowed to work near foods and should always use disposable, single use tissues when blowing your nose, coughing or sneezing. The mouth harbours *Staphylococci* bacteria and sweets, gum etc., should not be chewed by food handlers whilst on duty, nor should fingers be used for tasting, nor should food handlers' breath be used to 'polish' glassware etc.

*Spitting is a disgusting habit and is, in fact, illegal on food premises*

    Any food handler suffering from discharges from, ears, nose or eyes can contaminate food and they must report such discharges to their superior who must not allow them to handle food until they are medically authorised to do so.

## SMOKING

Smoking cigarettes, cigars, pipes or using snuff in food rooms or while you are handling open food is *illegal*
This is because:

◆    Whilst smoking you are touching your mouth and harmful bacteria, such as *Staphylococci* can be passed to the food

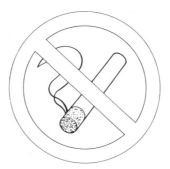

◆ Smoking encourages you to cough and sneeze

◆ Cigarette ends and ash may drop into the food causing contamination

◆ Cigarette ends, which are contaminated by saliva are placed on work surfaces encouraging cross-contamination

## WEARING OF JEWELLERY, PERFUME AND AFTERSHAVE etc.

Wearing aftershave and perfume by foods handlers should be discouraged as the food are quite likely to be tainted, especially those with a high fat content, causing contamination and complaints.

Earrings, watches, brooches, ornate finger rings etc., are positive dirt traps, where food particles and dust can collect and spread harmful bacteria and also cause skin diseases. Stones and metal can become dislodged from jewellery and be lost in the food, only to be 'found' by customers who always suffer damage to expensive dental work! It can also cause spoilage and contamination of the food. The only jewellery which should be allowed to be worn by food handlers is a gold wedding band.

## PROTECTIVE CLOTHING

The word protective is used in relation to the *food* and not you. It is the *food* which the protective clothing is protecting from outside sources of contamination! Dust, pet hairs, woollen fibres etc., are all likely to be found on outdoor clothes which can lead to contamination of food if they are allowed to be worn within the food areas. It is a requirement of the food handling regulations that all food handlers should wear *clean, washable, light-coloured protective clothing, with no external pockets and preferably with 'non-button type' fasteners.*

◆ If your protective clothing is worn *over* your outdoor clothing (not a very hygienic practice), it should completely cover all outdoor clothing, including sleeves, cuffs, collars etc

◆ Through contact with the air outside the food areas, ordinary clothing carries many harmful bacteria which can be spread by contact with equipment, work surfaces, hands, door handles etc., and so lead to cross-contamination

- External pockets are discouraged as they are likely to catch on machinery and also used to keep unhygienic articles etc

- Button-type fasteners are also discouraged as there is a possibility of them finding their way into the food and causing physical contamination

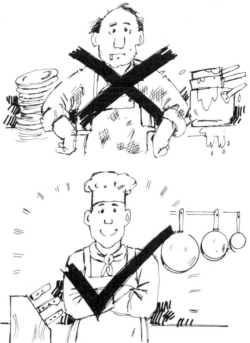

## GENERAL HEALTH CARE AND REPORTING OF ILLNESS

All food handlers have a *legal obligation* to inform their superiors if they are suffering from any illness which is likely to cause contamination of food stuffs and so food poisoning (vomiting, diarrhoea) or a food-borne illness.

If you are suffering from any illness such as described above then you must not be allowed to handle food until you are cleared by a medical certificate from your doctor, stating that you are fit to resume food–handling duties.

Any food handler who has eaten a meal known to have caused food poisoning, *or* lives in the household of a confirmed sufferer of food poisoning, *or* has suffered from vomiting and diarrhoea whilst abroad must not resume food handling duties without medical clearance.

# HYGIENE EDUCATION

## PREVENTION IS BETTER THAN CURE

It is always better to prevent the possibility of food poisoning, spoilage or contamination rather than having to cure actual outbreaks. This is best done by making sure that all staff are thoroughly educated and trained in the basic requirements of good hygiene practices *before* they are allowed to begin their duties. This basic training and instruction should then be followed up on a regular basis with refresher courses and meetings.

*Now complete the following questions at your own pace. When you have completed the questions, check your answers by reading through Section 3 again. Mark your answers using the answer grid at the end of package*

**I**   Complete the following list of occasions when a food handler should wash their hands.

*a*   after using the __.

*b*   in between handling ___ and _____ foods.

*c*   after _____ their hair.

*d*   on _____ the food preparation area and before using equipment or _____ any ____.

*e*   after eating, _____ or _____ their nose.

*f*   after handling _____ or waste food.

**2** In all cases of food poisoning, the main cause is human.      TRUE/FALSE

**3** Good standards of *personal hygiene* can help to reduce outbreaks of food poisoning.      TRUE/FALSE

**4** When should you, as a food handler, wash your hands?

  *a* at regular intervals throughout the day
  *b* after using the toilet
  *c* before beginning work
  *d* throughout the working day after each activity

**5** What should be used to cover a cut if you are working with food to protect against contamination?

  *a* sterile dressing
  *b* flesh coloured dressing
  *c* coloured dressing
  *d* waterproof, coloured dressing

**6** Which bacteria thrives in the nose, throat and mouth?

  *a* *Salmonella*
  *b* *Staphylococci*
  *c* *Clostridium*
  *d* *Listeria*

**7** Why is smoking illegal in food premises?

  *a* smoke and cigarette ash are unpleasant to others
  *b* smoking involves contact with the mouth and encourages cross – contamination
  *c* smoking is considered contributory to cancer
  *d* cigarette ends can find their way into food

**8** Food handlers protective clothing must be

  *a* clean
  *b* made of cotton
  *c* freshly ironed
  *d* white

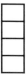

**9**    Why must protective clothing be worn by food handlers?

    *a*  to give a clean, hygienic appearance
    *b*  to protect the food handler from harmful bacteria
    *c*  to protect food from harmful bacteria
    *d*  to prevent food handlers clothing becoming dirty

**10**    You report for work after being ill overnight with diarrhoea. What should you do?

    *a*  take an aspirin every 4 hours
    *b*  report to sick bay
    *c*  wash your hands more often than usual
    *d*  report it to your supervisor

# SECTION FOUR

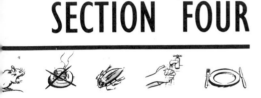

# *Bacteria – what are they?*

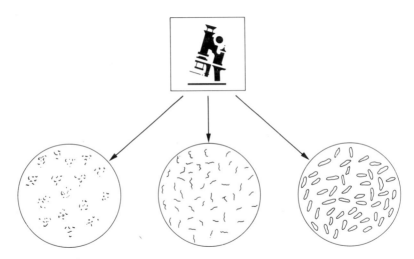

***Fig. 4.1*** *Looking through a microscope at bacteria*

Bacteria are microscopic organisms which are found everywhere, on man, in water, in soil and in the air we breathe, and are not visible to the naked eye. The majority of bacteria are quite harmless, in fact some are essential in breaking down decaying matter and in the production of cheese and yogurt.

There are harmful bacteria which cause food spoilage and some, known as pathogens, which are responsible for causing illness. The bacteria which we shall be concentrating on are the harmful bacteria which, when allowed to multiply, result in food poisoning. Each of these harmful bacteria will be discussed in parts a, b and c of this section. It is the number of these harmful bacteria present in food which can be used to determine whether or not the food has been handled correctly.

When raw meat is prepared for stews, pies sausages etc., it is minced, diced or cubed and this involves a lot of handling which allows the bacteria normally on the surface of the food to be 'mixed' in and so spread throughout the food.

# Conditions for growing bacteria

Bacteria are exactly the same as other forms of life when it comes to the requirements they need to multiply and grow. These requirements are: *WARMTH; FOOD; MOISTURE* and *TIME.* Under all these conditions one bacteria can multiply to become sixteen million (16,000,000) bacteria within eight hours!

Good hygiene practices are therefore absolutely *essential* to stop this growth cycle.

## WARMTH

Food poisoning bacteria thrive (from 1 to 16,000,000 in 8 hours) at a temperature of 37°C which is the normal body temperature. At temperatures between 5°C and 65°C bacteria are capable of multiplying at a considerable rate. Outside this temperature range bacteria multiplication is greatly reduced; at 100°C bacteria are killed, and below 0°C all bacterial growth is retarded. If you are to control the multiplication and growth rate of bacteria it is obvious that you must control the temperature at which foods are stored and cooked. The temperature at which food should be kept to control and prevent growth is:

*BELOW 5°C*

*or*

*ABOVE 65°C*

The temperature range between 5°C and 65°C is quite rightly known as the *DANGER ZONE* (see Fig. 4.2).

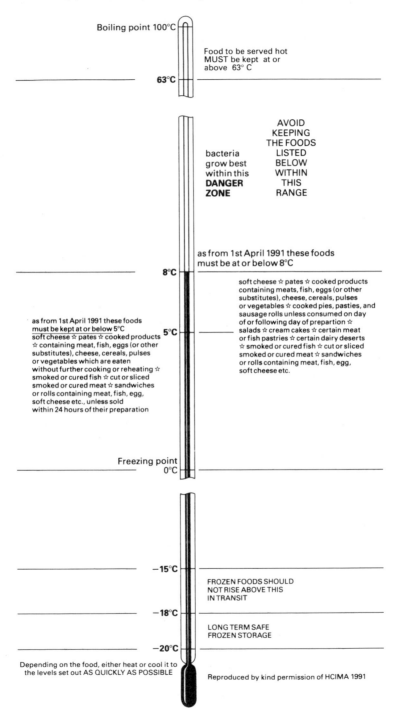

FOOD HYGIENE (AMENDED) REGULATIONS 1990

Boiling point 100°C

Food to be served hot
MUST be kept at or
above 63° C

63°C

AVOID
KEEPING
THE FOODS
bacteria          LISTED
grow best         BELOW
within this       WITHIN
**DANGER**        THIS
**ZONE**          RANGE

as from 1st April 1991 these foods
must be at or below 8°C

8°C

soft cheese ☆ pates ☆ cooked products
containing meats, fish, eggs (or other
substitutes), cheese, cereals, pulses
or vegetables ☆ cooked pies, pasties, and
sausage rolls unless consumed on day
as from 1st April 1991 these foods         of or following day of prepartion ☆
must be kept at or below 5°C               salads ☆ cream cakes ☆ certain meat
soft cheese ☆ pates ☆ cooked products     or fish pastries ☆ certain dairy deserts
☆ containing meat, fish, eggs (or other    ☆ smoked or cured fish ☆ cut or sliced
substitutes), cheese, cereals, pulses      smoked or cured meat ☆ sandwiches
or vegetables which are eaten              or rolls containing meat, fish, egg,
without further cooking or reheating ☆     soft cheese etc.
smoked or cured fish ☆ cut or sliced
smoked or cured meat ☆ sandwiches

5°C

or rolls containing meat, fish, egg,
soft cheese etc., unless sold
within 24 hours of their preparation

Freezing point
0°C

−15°C

FROZEN FOODS SHOULD
NOT RISE ABOVE THIS
IN TRANSIT

−18°C

LONG TERM SAFE
FROZEN STORAGE

−20°C

Depending on the food, either heat or cool it to
the levels set out AS QUICKLY AS POSSIBLE        Reproduced by kind permission of HCIMA 1991

**Fig. 4.2**  *Diagram showing the 'Danger Zone' (5°C–65°C)*

Making sure that food is kept outside the *danger zone* does not prevent all bacteria multiplication, as some bacteria are capable of producing *spores* which enable them to survive even higher/lower temperatures.

## FOOD & MOISTURE

Bacteria prefer foods with a high protein content such as cooked meat, poultry and dairy produce (known as *high risk foods*). Dried egg and milk do not hold any attraction to bacteria until they are diluted with water, when any bacteria present will begin growing – any such foods should then be treated as fresh and used as quickly as possible after reconstitution and stored in a refrigerator.

Foods which have a high concentration of sugar, salt, acid or other preservatives do not support bacterial growth. As well as food, most bacteria also require moist surroundings and it is generally the case that food preparation areas contain both these essential ingredients for supporting bacterial growth and so great care and attention must be given to the storage, preparation and cooking of food.

## TIME

If you give bacteria the right conditions of food, moisture and warmth, some can divide into two every 10–20 minutes. This division is known as *binary fission*. The diagram below shows how this happens.

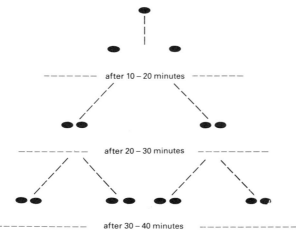

*Fig. 4.3* *Diagram showing how bacteria divide and multiply*

If sufficient time is allowed, a very small number of single bacteria can multiply to such an extent that there are enough to cause *food poisoning*. It is therefore *essential* that foods known as *high risk foods* are not left within the *danger zone* for any longer than is absolutely necessary.

*Now complete the following questions at your own pace. When you have completed the questions, check your answers by reading through Section 4 again. Mark your answers using the answer grid at the end of package*

**1** Food poisoning is caused by

*a* the number of bacteria found on food
*b* all bacteria found on food
*c* a single bacterium found on food
*d* a combination of bacteria found on food

**2** In order to multiply, bacteria need which conditions?

| | | | |
|---|---|---|---|
| *a* Food | Space | Warmth | Moisture |
| *b* Food | Time | Warmth | Moisture |
| *c* Food | Light | Warmth | Moisture |
| *d* Food | Air | Warmth | Moisture |

**3** At which temperature do bacteria multiply most rapidly?

*a* 5°C
*b* 65°C
*c* 100°C
*d* 37°C

**4** The DANGER ZONE is within which temperature range?

*a* 5°C–35°C
*b* 5°C–45°C
*c* 5°C–55°C
*d* 5°C–65°C

**5** In ideal conditions bacteria can divide into 2 every 10–20 minutes. What do you call this method of reproduction?

B _ _ _ _ Y _ _ S _ _ _ N

**6** At which of the following temperatures would bacteria be killed?

*a*   0°C
*b*   37°C
*c*   65°C
*d*   100°C

# *Introducing Salmonella, Clostridium, Staphylococcus*

With names like that its no wonder we want to wipe them off the face of the earth! Don't bother too much about remembering the names of the bacteria, but concentrate more on the way the bacteria grow and multiply and the ways in which you can *control* the growth and multiplication rate.

In the rest of this section (a, b and c) we will take each bacteria and look at it in a little more detail.

◆ We will look at the *onset time/incubation period* – this is the time between eating the food and the first signs of illness

◆ We will look at the *duration of illness* – this is the length of time that you would normally suffer from the illness

◆ We will look at the *symptoms* – these are the signs which show you are suffering from the illness

◆ We will look at the ways in which we can *prevent* food poisoning caused by these bacteria

## SECTION FOUR A  *Salmonella*

The *Salmonella* bacteria cause approx 70% of reported cases of food poisoning. There are about 20–40 fatal cases of *Salmonella* food poisoning every year, usually in the very young, sick or elderly.

**Onset time:**        6–72 hours

**Duration of illness:**    11–18 days

**Symptoms:**        *Diarrhoea, headaches, fever and abdominal pain*

*Salmonella* bacteria are found in the intestines of man and animal and on the fur and feet of pests such as rats, mice and flies. *Salmonella* poisoning is usually caused by:

◆ Eating uncooked foods . . . such as untreated milk

◆ Eating undercooked or partially thawed foods

◆ Cross – contamination

*Salmonella* can be brought into the food area on the surface of raw foods such as meat, poultry and sausages and the shells of eggs. It is found in the centre of poultry and widely distributed within 'made-up' dishes such as pies, casseroles etc. If the food is not cooked and stored correctly the bacteria present begin growing and multiplying and so can cause an outbreak of food poisoning quite easily. The organisms are spread by cross-contamination from raw to cooked foods by, for example, using the same chopping boards or knives for both raw and cooked foods without correct disinfection between tasks.

A common cause of cross-contamination is from the handlers' clothing: if they do not wear separate protective clothing *or* wear their protective clothing for duties outside the food areas – for example, popping to the shops to get a newspaper, wearing their protective clothing to travel to and from work.

Insects, birds and domestic pets can spread *salmonella* into food if they are allowed into food areas, by contact with surfaces etc., or by handlers stroking pets and immediately returning to food preparation duties without washing their hands with bactericidal soap.

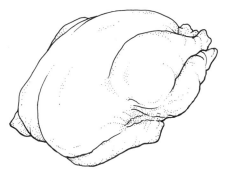

**Fig. 4.4**  *'Handle with care – ready-packed Salmonella!'*

*Salmonella* are easily killed by heat and so many cases of food poisoning are caused by inadequately cooked foods and cross-contamination of foods after they have been cooked.

**Great care must always be taken when dealing with poultry of any kind as it is estimated that 80% of all poultry is contaminated with *SALMONELLA*.**

## *Preventing Salmonella poisoning*

◆ Cook food thoroughly, making sure that the centre of the food is at sufficiently high a temperature to kill all bacteria. (The use of a digital-probe thermometer is ideal for this purpose.)

◆ Thaw frozen foods completely before cooking, especially poultry. Always thaw poultry in a refrigerator and *not* under warm running water in a sink. (A large turkey may take as long as 48 hours to thaw completely.)

◆ Have separate boards and knives for the preparation of raw and cooked foods to avoid the risk of cross-contamination from the surface of the raw foods

◆ Always clean and disinfect equipment thoroughly after use and before beginning another process. (Mincing raw chicken livers for pâté and then immediately mincing raw vegetables for cornish pasties without disinfecting the mincer is an *ideal recipe* for food poisoning.)

◆ You should have separate refrigerators for the storage of raw and cooked foods (especially meats). If this is not possible you should always store raw meats on the bottom shelf of the fridge so that blood cannot drip onto cooked foods and so contaminate them. NEVER store dairy foods, custards, trifles etc., in the same fridge as raw meats, fish or poultry

◆ Wash your hands thoroughly after handling raw and cooked foods, especially poultry

◆ Keep foods out of the *danger zone* to prevent multiplication of bacteria and pay particular attention to the temperature of stews, gravies etc., which are kept hot during service times

◆ Do not eat untreated foods such as 'green top' milk

*Now complete the following questions at your own pace. When you have completed the questions, check your answers by reading through Section 4A again. Mark your answers using the answer grid at the end of package*

I   Fill in the missing words in the following statements.

   *a*   _____ ____/_____ ____ this is the time between eating the food and the first signs of illness.

   *b*   _____ __ _____ this is the length of time that you would normally suffer from the illness.

   *c*   _____ these are the signs which show you are suffering from the illness.

**2** Which one of the following would be most likely to cause *Salmonella* food poisoning?

   *a*   dried milk powder
   *b*   pickled eggs
   *c*   chicken
   *d*   sultanas

**3** Domestic pets are a source of *Salmonella* bacteria.       TRUE/FALSE

**4** Eating undercooked or partially thawed foods can cause *Salmonella* food poisoning.       TRUE/FALSE

**5** Many cases of *Salmonella* food poisoning are caused by incorrectly thawing poultry.       TRUE/FALSE

## SECTION FOUR B *Clostridium*

*Clostridium*, or more correctly, *Clostridium perfringens*, is responsible for approx 20% of all reported cases of food poisoning every year.

| | |
|---|---|
| **Onset time:** | 8–22 hours. |
| **Duration of illness:** | 12–48 hours. |
| **Symptoms:** | *Abdominal pains, diarrhoea, vomiting is rare.* |

*Clostridium perfringens* grows best in the absence of oxygen and is usually found in stock pots, the bottom of stews or in the centre of large masses of food, particularly rolled meat joints such as rolled brisket, breast of lamb etc. It is also found in the intestines of man and animals, and flies and bluebottles are usually heavily infected.

    *Clostridium perfringens* can form *spores*. A spore is best described as a hard shell which the bacteria forms around itself enabling it to withstand extremes of temperature. When the temperature is ideal for growth (within the danger zone) the outer shell is dissolved and growth and multiplication begin again. The spores of *Clostridium perfringens* are found in soil and the soil dust from vegetables, sacks etc., can contaminate food if it is allowed to settle after being brought into the food areas (often on the protective clothing of food handlers).

The spores of *clostridium perfringens* are *not* destroyed by cooking and can withstand boiling, stewing, steaming for up to 5 hours.

The spores do not multiply unless the food is allowed to stand or is kept warm within the *danger zone* for any length of time before serving. They then germinate, producing bacteria which multiply rapidly within this temperature range.

## *Preventing Clostridium perfringens poisoning*

◆ Always have separate *preparation areas* for raw and cooked foods, especially meat and vegetables

◆ Always have separate boards and knives for the preparation of raw and cooked foods

◆ Always clean and disinfect equipment thoroughly after use and before beginning another process

◆ Store raw and cooked foods separately

◆ Cool cooked foods rapidly and refrigerate immediately after cooling. It is advisable to divide large quantities of food into small units in order to allow rapid cooling. Always break down large joints of meat into units of 2½–3 kilos for cooking so that they will cool down quicker. Always remove meats from any cooking liquor immediately after cooking to allow rapid cooling

◆ Wash your hands thoroughly after handling raw meat and unwashed vegetables

◆ Try never to re-heat food, but if it is necessary make sure that it is brought to a temperature of 100°C as quickly as possible and serve it immediately. Never re-heat foods, especially meats more than once. The best method of re-heating foods quickly is to use a microwave oven (at the correct time and temperature settings) or by deep frying

## *MICROWAVE COOKERY*

**The food is heated from the inside to the outside.** When you use a microwave cooker you are re-heating by means of rays which penetrate the food and cause the molecules within the food to agitate or move. This movement causes friction between the molecules and causes heat to be generated. It is this heat which re-heats the foods, and because it is generated at the centre of the food it is the most reliable method of thoroughly heating foods to the temperature required.

Under normal cooking methods the heat is applied to the outside of the food first and it is possible for the food to appear cooked when in fact the centre is only warm and therefore liable to bacterial growth and multiplication. It is essential that the timing of the microwave is calculated carefully as the time needed to efficiently heat the foods thoroughly depends on the volume or mass of the food being heated.

'Cold spots' (pockets of food which do not reach the required temperature to kill bacteria) in the food are likely if such attention is not given to the timing. The more food that is placed into the microwave, the more time will be needed to completely cook or re-heat the food at that temperature setting.

> **Microwave ovens are not 'magic boxes'**

## *DEEP FRYING*

Deep frying is another very quick, high temperature method of cookery and is used to re-heat or cook, small, tender pieces of food. The temperature of the oil is usually at 180°C and can penetrate to the centre of the food very quickly and so makes sure that the food is thoroughly cooked or heated to the centre.

*Now complete the
following questions at your own pace.
When you have completed the questions, check your
answers by reading through Section 4B again.
Mark your answers using the
answer grid at the end
of package*

**1** Stew, stock and sauces are particularly prone to *clostridium* food poisoning. TRUE/FALSE

**2** *Clostridium* bacteria can produce 'shells' around themselves which are able to withstand extremes of temperature. These are known as

   *a* Pathogens
   *b* Viruses
   *c* Spores
   *d* Carriers

**3** The soil and dirt which sticks to vegetables carries *clostridium* bacteria. TRUE/FALSE

**4** You should always cool foods as quickly as possible after cooking to prevent the possibility of *clostridium* food poisoning. TRUE/FALSE

**5** The cooking time for foods cooked through a microwave oven is decided by the mass or volume of the food to be cooked. TRUE/FALSE

**6** Foods which have been cooked through a microwave oven should be allowed to stand for approx 1 minute before serving so that:

   *a* they are cool enough to handle easily

**b** cold spots in the food can reach a safe temperature which prevents bacterial growth □

**c** to allow the oven to gain correct temperature
**d** reduce shrinkage of the food ⊟

**7** All foods cooked through a microwave oven are completely safe to eat. TRUE/FALSE

## SECTION FOUR C  *Staphylococcus*

*Staphylococcus* or *Staphylococcus aureus*, to give it its correct name, is responsible for about 4% of all reported cases of food poisoning every year. The symptoms are severe for a short period but food poisoning from *Staphylococcus aureus* is rarely fatal.

| | |
|---|---|
| **Onset time:** | 2–6 hours |
| **Duration of illness:** | 6–24 hours. |
| **Symptoms:** | *Vomiting, abdominal pains.* |

*Staphylococcus aureus* is often found in the nose, throat and on the hands of healthy people. It is present around septic cuts, spots, boils, styes and grazes. *Staphylococcus aureus* is not easily removed from the hands by washing and when it grows on food it produces a *toxin*. The organism itself is destroyed by cooking but the toxins are more resistant. *Staphylococcus aureus* is spread by food handlers who sneeze, cough over food, or who have cuts, boils etc., and do not cover them with clean waterproof, coloured dressings. Staff suffering from vomiting, diarrhoea, throat or skin infections who continue to work with food can spread *Staphylococcus* bacteria.

## *Preventing Staphylococcus poisoning*

◆ Maintain high stands of personal hygiene and make sure that all staff follow good hygiene practices

◆ Handle food as little as possible. Use tongs, forks, plastic gloves where ever possible to reduce actual hand contact with the food. This is especially important with food which will not be heated again before serving

**Remember: washing your hands does not remove all *Staphylococci* from them**

◆ Keep foods as cold as possible to reduce the rate of multiplication of bacteria

◆ *Never* use fingers to 'taste' food during preparation and always disinfect cutlery etc., which is used for tasting immediately after use

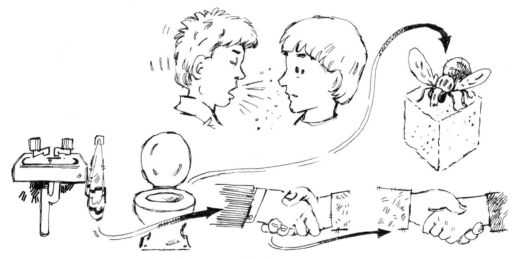

**Fig. 4.5** *Methods of spreading Staphylococcus aureus*

*Now complete the*
*following questions at your own pace.*
*When you have completed the questions, check your*
*answers by reading through Section 4C again.*
*Mark your answers using the*
*answer grid at the end*
*of package*

1   *Staphylococcus* food poisoning can be caused by excessive handling of
    foods.                                                    TRUE/FALSE

2   All traces of *Staphylococcus* can be removed from your hands by
    thorough washing.                                         TRUE/FALSE

3   High standards of personal hygiene helps to reduce levels of
    *Staphylococcus* bacteria.                                TRUE/FALSE

4   *Staphylococcus* bacteria can be transferred onto food stuffs if you fail to
    cover cuts etc. with waterproof coloured dressings.       TRUE/FALSE

5   Which one of the following would be the safest way to handle fresh
    cream eclairs?

    *a*   clean hands
    *b*   clean pair of tongs
    *c*   a clean fork
    *d*   a clean spoon

6   Which of the following would cause *staphylococcus* bacteria to
    contaminate foodstuffs?

    *a*   using colour coded boards
    *b*   coughing in the kitchen
    *c*   cooling foods as quickly as possible
    *d*   using a waterproof, coloured dressing on a cut

# SECTION FIVE

# *What is food poisoning?*

Food poisoning is a very unpleasant illness which usually occurs within 1–36 hours of eating *contaminated* or *poisonous food*. Symptoms usually last for 1–7 days and include one or more of the following: *NAUSEA, VOMITING, ABDOMINAL PAIN, DIARRHOEA*.

Food poisoning is caused by:

Bacteria or their poisons

Viruses

Chemicals

Metals

Poisonous plants

*Bacterial food poisoning* is the most common of these and in some cases can cause death.

Food poisoning is caused by *ignorance* or *negligence* and therefore it is widely accepted that a reduction in the current statistics can only be achieved by the *education and training* of food handlers in efficient food hygiene standards. One mistake by an untrained food handler in even the most modern and hygienic premises can result in an outbreak of food poisoning. The principles of food hygiene must be taught in a logical and professional manner as an essential part of initial training. (Preferably before the food handler actually begins his employment.) No food handler should be allowed to touch food until they have successfully completed a basic course of hygiene instruction.

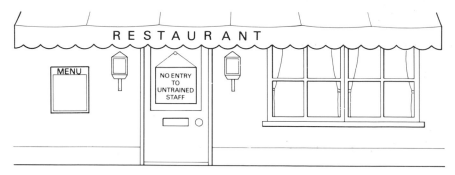

Good hygiene practices should become a 'way of life' to all food handlers and so be practised and perfected throughout the food industry.

# Points to remember about food poisoning

◆ Foods which cause food poisoning, look, taste and smell normal

◆ Food poisoning bacteria are everywhere

◆ The main reason for food poisoning is the storage of *high risk foods* at room temperature

◆ Given warmth, time and food and moisture, harmful bacteria multiply rapidly

◆ Loss of business, jobs and life are the result of the many thousands of cases of food poisoning which occur annually

# Main reasons for food poisoning

◆ Food prepared too far in advance and stored within the *danger zone* rather than in a refrigerator

◆ Cooling foods too slowly before refrigeration

◆ Not re-heating foods to the correct temperature in order to destroy food poisoning bacteria

◆ The use of cooked food which is contaminated with food poisoning bacteria

◆ Undercooking of foods

◆ Not thawing frozen poultry and meat for sufficient time or in the wrong manner

◆ Cross-contamination between raw and cooked foods during preparation and storage

◆ Storing hot foods below 65°C

◆ Infected food handlers

◆ Incorrect and careless use of leftovers

◆ Cross-contamination due to ignorance and carelessness in cleaning techniques

## *Food-borne diseases*

So far in this training package we have discussed food poisoning and found that bacteria must be given time, food and moisture and warmth so that they can grow and multiply and produce sufficient bacteria to cause an outbreak of *food poisoning.*

There are other illnesses which can be transmitted through food and these are known as *food-borne diseases.*

These diseases are caused through bacteria and viruses but *only require small numbers* to cause illness. Such diseases are:

*Typhoid, Paratyphoid, Dysentery* and *Brucellosis.*

The bacteria responsible for food-borne diseases are found in man's intestines and the *chain of infection* follows the same cycle as that for food poisoning.

**BACTERIA IN FAECES**
↓
**transferred via hands**
↓
**ON TO THE FOOD**
↓
**food is consumed**
↓
**ILLNESS IS CAUSED**

*Now complete the
following questions at your own pace.
When you have completed the questions, check your
answers by reading through Section 5 again.
Mark your answers using the
answer grid at the end
of package*

**1**   Premises which are clean and tidy do not harbour food poisoning
      bacteria.                                                  TRUE/FALSE

**2**   Which of the following symptoms would indicate that you could be
      suffering from food poisoning?

      *a*  fever and sore throat
      *b*  nausea and headaches
      *c*  diarrhoea and stomach pains
      *d*  fever and headaches

**3**   Which of the following cause most outbreaks of food poisoning?

      *a*  microwave cookery
      *b*  food prepared too far in advance of requirements
      *c*  pest infestation
      *d*  using incorrect cleaning procedures

**4**   Food poisoning is only caused by harmful bacteria.       TRUE/FALSE

**5**   Incorrect storage of *high risk foods* leads to many outbreaks of food
      poisoning                                                  TRUE/FALSE

# SECTION SIX

# Preventing food poisoning

Before we begin this section we should take time to understand a combination of foods which are particularly at risk from bacterial contamination. These are known as *HIGH RISK FOODS*. Care has to be taken with *all* food in order to reduce the possibility of contamination and outbreaks of food poisoning.

*High risk foods* are those which are intended for consumption without additional cooking or preservation, which would normally destroy the harmful bacteria. Such foods are usually high protein foods which require refrigerated storage.

◆ *All cooked meat and poultry items*

*Cooked meat products* – pies, sausages, pâtés etc.

*Gravies, stews and stocks*

*Egg products* – mayonnaise, egg custards etc.

*Milk, cream and all dairy products* – including ice cream

*Cooked rice*

*Shellfish and other seafood*

*SPECIAL ATTENTION MUST BE GIVEN TO THE STORAGE OF HIGH RISK FOODS*

*High risk foods* are nearly always implicated in food poisoning outbreaks, particularly poultry and poultry products, although food poisoning does not necessarily result from eating these products alone. The foods which cause food poisoning do not need to exhibit any obvious signs of contamination either in taste, sight or smell. Extreme care and control is therefore essential to prevent contamination and bacterial multiplication.

---

**It is a legal requirement that all cases or suspected cases of food poisoning are reported to the Local Environmental Health Officer for investigation.**

---

The number of cases which are reported is estimated to be only 10% of the total number of actual cases of food poisoning. In the past 10 years the number of reported cases has, in general, risen and an average of 10,000–15,000 cases are reported annually. This means that in fact there is estimated to be 100,000–150,000 cases of food poisoning every year!

Take a few minutes to think about why there has been such a dramatic increase in the number of food poisoning incidences and jot down your reasons on a piece of paper.

Now check your reasons with those given below. Instances of food poisoning have increased in recent years because of:

◆ Public awareness of the dangers of incorrect handling of foodstuffs which leads to bacteria growth and potential food poisoning outbreaks

◆ Increased consumption of ready-prepared and convenience foods which only require 'warming up' before eating

◆ Increased eating out, both at work and socially – take away restaurants, sandwich bars etc.

◆ Shopping being done weekly rather than daily and kept in car boots, warm lockers etc., for long periods which encourages bacterial growth

◆ Changes in catering techniques to reduce staff numbers employed – especially equipment for reheating foods prior to serving

◆ Much wider media coverage of outbreaks which leads to greater consumer awareness

◆ Extensive national distribution of food products due to road, rail and air network

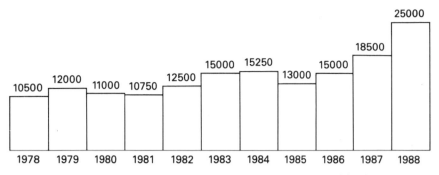

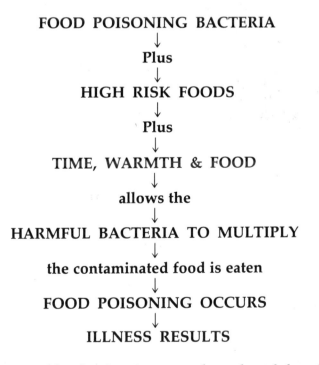

**Fig. 6.1**  *How the annual number of reported incidences of food poisoning have increased in England and Wales from 1978–1988 (in general terms)*

Food poisoning, like accidents, does not just *happen*, it is *caused*. Food poisoning is caused by a chain of events taking place, all of which can be prevented.

**FOOD POISONING BACTERIA**
↓
**Plus**
↓
**HIGH RISK FOODS**
↓
**Plus**
↓
**TIME, WARMTH & FOOD**
↓
**allows the**
↓
**HARMFUL BACTERIA TO MULTIPLY**
↓
**the contaminated food is eaten**
↓
**FOOD POISONING OCCURS**
↓
**ILLNESS RESULTS**

If the cases of food poisoning are to be reduced then it is essential that the *chain of events* leading to the illness is broken.

*HOW DO YOU DO THAT?*

There are three main ways in which this chain of events can be broken.

**PROTECT** *the food from contamination*
**PREVENT** *bacteria multiplication in the food*
**DESTROY** *bacteria present in the food*

# How can you protect the food from contamination?

◆ Maintain the highest possible standards of personal hygiene

◆ Make sure that all food handlers wear the correct protective clothing and follow rules regarding wearing of jewellery, perfumes etc.

◆ Only handle glassware, plates, cutlery etc. by those parts which do not come into contact with food – stems, rims, handles etc. Do *not* polish glasses, plates and cutlery by *breathing* on them

◆ Follow the correct methods for cleaning food preparation and production areas

◆ Always keep food and equipment off the floor at all times

◆ Do not use dirty, or insufficiently cleaned equipment and knives

◆ Do not use wash hand basins for washing food and equipment, nor wash your hands in food preparation sinks

◆ Remove all waste and swill immediately to a raised, covered container, well away from the food area

◆ Make sure that liquid from thawed frozen foods, especially poultry, does not come into contact with *high risk* foods, surfaces or equipment used for the preparation of high risk foods

◆ Keep all foods covered where ever possible. Store food in containers which have tight fitting lids to prevent access by rodents and insects

◆ Only handle food when it is absolutely necessary – use tongs, forks, trays, plates etc., rather than hands. Use disposable surgical type gloves when excessive handling of food is necessary – sandwiches, retail display etc.

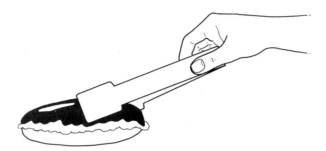

**Fig. 6.2**   *Handling cream cakes the correct way*

◆   Keep raw and cooked foods separate throughout *storage, preparation, cooking and serving*

◆   Make sure that you have separate surfaces and knives for the preparation of raw and *high risk foods*

◆   Do not use dirty or soiled cloths in the food area for drying or cleaning processes

◆   Do not let domestic pets into the food area and make sure that rodents and insects are not encouraged

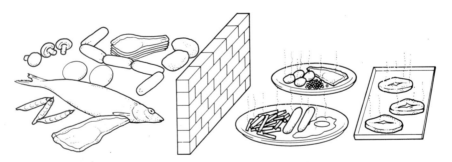

**Fig. 6.3**   *Keep cooked food and raw food apart from each other*

## How can you prevent bacteria multiplication in the food?

◆   Always be aware of the *danger zone* and store foods below 5°C or above 65°C

◆   When preparing foods make sure that they are in the *danger zone* for as short a time as possible. Food should be cooked or refrigerated as soon as they have been prepared, not left on the bench, at room temperature and above, allowing bacteria to multiply and grow

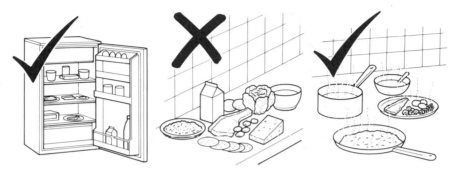

**Fig. 6.4** *The right and wrong way to prepare food*

◆ Make sure that dried goods are stored correctly to stop them absorbing moisture

◆ Make full use of methods of preservation to reduce bacteria multiplication

# *Preservation*

> **It is essential to realise that foods which are protected by preservation must be handled with as much care and consideration as fresh foods, especially once they have been opened, thawed, diluted etc. Then they must be kept in refrigerated conditions as they are just as likely to attract bacterial growth as normal, fresh products.**

Preservation is carried out on foods to reduce the risk of contamination and bacterial growth. Some methods of preservation do not alter the food a great deal, whereas other methods do change the food flavours, appearance and nutritional values quite a lot. All methods of preservation are designed purely to stop the bacterial growth within the foods and so make them safer to use and easier to store without being contaminated.

## METHODS OF PRESERVATION

**Freezing**   this is where foods are taken to a temperature of −18°C by various means and at this temperature all bacterial growth is retarded.

**Drying**   this is where all or part of the moisture is removed from foods and, as you now know, bacteria require moisture to live and so this again retards the bacterial growth.

**Canning**   when foods are canned or bottled they are sterilised and this sterilisation kills all harmful bacteria present.

**Preserving in syrup, sugar, salt or vinegar**   any food which contains a high percentage of sugar, salt or acid, such as vinegar does not attract bacterial growth and therefore if it is kept in correct storage conditions is less likely to cause multiplication of bacteria.

**Pasteurisation and sterilisation**   foods which have been pasteurised or undergone any other method of heat treatment will have had all harmful bacteria in that food killed.

**Vacuum-packing**   foods which are vacuum-packed have been sealed in containers which have had all the air or oxygen removed. Bacteria need oxygen to multiply and grow and so their growth rate is retarded while the food is vacuum packed.

# How can you destroy bacteria present within food?

As you will have realised by going through this training package so far, everything has bacteria on it. Some of the bacteria are harmless, but others can cause food spoilage and food poisoning. In order to reduce outbreaks of food poisoning and cases of food spoilage these bacteria have to be destroyed. You will also have found out that it is a combination of time and temperature controls which prevent bacterial growth and multiplication. Applying heat to most foods, will destroy all bacteria within the food. Therefore the correct and thorough cooking of food will destroy bacteria.

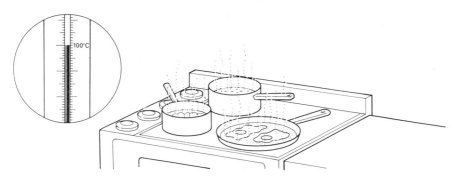

**Fig. 6.5** *The correct temperature for cooking food*

By applying other forms of heat treatment to food will destroy bacteria.

By 'other forms of heat treatment' we mean sterilisation, pasteurisation, canning etc.

> **It is essential to remember also that some bacteria can produce *spores* which are heat resistant and germinate when conditions are favourable. The correct storage of such foods after cooking etc is important if these spores are to be controlled and not allowed to grow and multiply.**

*Now complete the
following questions at your own pace.
When you have completed the questions, check your
answers by reading through Section 6 again.
Mark your answers using the
answer grid at the end
of package*

**I**   Which of the following statements is correct?

    *a*  contaminated food looks, smells, feels and tastes normal
    *b*  cooking food makes it safe from contamination
    *c*  frozen chicken is best thawed under warm water
    *d*  washing equipment makes it bacteria free

**2**   Which of the following would be classed as *'high risk foods'*?

    *a*  Dried Milk   Lentils      Canned Fruit
    *b*  Fresh Steak  Fruit          Vegetables
    *c*  Kippers     Bacon         Jam
    *d*  Boiled Ham  Mayonnaise  Cheese

**3**   Waste food should be stored in

    *a*  metal containers
    *b*  plastic refuse sacks
    *c*  lidded containers
    *d*  plastic dustbins

**4**   Food can be protected from *contamination* by

    *a*  practising high standards of personal hygiene
    *b*  only using first class quality foodstuffs
    *c*  correct and thorough cooking of food
    *d*  providing wash and hand basins in food prep areas

**5**   Bacteria can be prevented from *multiplying* by

    *a*   using colour coded boards in kitchens
    *b*   not storing food within the danger zone
    *c*   using clean cloths for drying equipment
    *d*   using only first class quality foodstuffs

**6**   Harmful bacteria in food can be *destroyed* by

    *a*   thorough cooking of foods.
    *b*   storing raw and cooked foods separately.
    *c*   using colour coded boards in kitchens
    *d*   disinfecting all surfaces in food area

# SECTION SEVEN

# Food contamination

All the way through this training package you will have come across the word: CONTAMINATION.

The whole aim of your learning good hygiene standards and practices is so that you can reduce the cases of contamination and so make food more safe to eat. Contamination has already been defined at the beginning of the pack as:

*the presence of any objectionable matter in food – either bacteria, metal, poison or anything which makes the food unsuitable for people to eat.*

This contamination is usually caused through *bacteria* but there are other things which contaminate food. Before we list the four types of contamination it is important to realise that most cases are caused by ignorance and carelessness on the part of the food handler!

## Sources of contamination

The four types of contamination are:

◆ Bacterial contamination

◆ Chemical contamination

◆ Natural or vegetable contamination

◆ Physical contamination

We will now look at each method of contamination in more detail.

# BACTERIAL CONTAMINATION

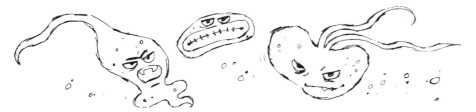

Bacterial contamination is the most common cause of food poisoning, and results from *ignorance and carelessness* on the part of the food handler than by any other reason. The *lack of facilities* to allow food handlers to operate high standards of food hygiene also contribute greatly to bacterial contamination. *Inadequate work space, storage facilities* (fridges etc.), *washing facilities* both for personnel and equipment all contribute to the many thousands of cases of cross contamination which result in food spoilage, poisoning and even death every year.

The *lack of refrigerator space* means that foods have to be left in warm, moist food areas for long periods of time which are the ideal conditions the bacteria are seeking to multiply and thrive.

The *lack of sufficient refrigeration* means that all sorts of foods: raw, cooked, dairy etc., are placed in one fridge and this allows food to be spilt, knocked and contaminated whilst being stored incorrectly.

# CHEMICAL CONTAMINATION

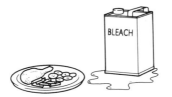

Chemical contamination is where the food is contaminated by chemicals either during growth, storage, preparation, cooking or packaging processes. While most cases of chemical contamination occur in the home or food manufacturing areas, great care must be taken to ensure that there are no chemicals (bleach, paraffin, caustics etc.) *anywhere* where food is being handled.

Chemicals should only be stored in the containers they are bought in and not transferred into other containers, such as lemonade bottles etc.

*Always* dispose of chemical containers safely, as soon as they are empty.

It is also possible to get chemical poisoning through metals, such as lead, by prolonged absorption through the body.

# Natural or vegetable contamination

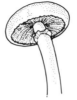

Natural or vegetable contamination is where plants, which are poisonous, are allowed to become 'confused' with or mixed together with otherwise 'clean' foods. Such things as toad-stools, hemlock, rhubarb leaves, berries, red kidney beans etc.

# Physical contamination

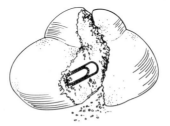

Physical contamination is where *foreign bodies* are allowed to become mixed with, or drop into, foods during storage, preparation or cooking. One very common cause of physical contamination happens when workmen, such as painters, plumbers etc., are working in food areas and the food is not covered correctly so allowing nuts, bolts etc., to fall into the food. Where machinery is used for certain processes in the food areas it is often found that stray parts become loose and fall into foods.

# Sources of bacteria causing contamination

*The person*   People have food poisoning bacteria in their mouth, nose, intestines and on their skin. *Direct* contamination can occur when they cough, sneeze or even whistle in the food areas. Similarly if food handlers do not wash their hands after using the W.C. direct contamination can take place. *Indirect* contamination occurs through the use of sewage-contaminated water.

All water used, for whatever purpose, in food premises must be suitably treated, i.e. *chlorination.*

The Aberdeen Typhoid (Food-borne disease) was caused by damaged cans of corned beef being cooled in sewage polluted water.

*Raw foods*   All raw foods are vehicles for contamination, especially red meat, poultry, shellfish and untreated milk. It is estimated that 80% of all poultry carry *Salmonella bacteria*!

The liquids from defrosting foods, especially poultry, must not be allowed to contaminate work surfaces, wiping cloths, uniform, chopping boards, equipment and particularly *high risk foods*.

> **Raw foods must be kept separate from *high risk foods*
> and cooked foods at all times.**

Soil contains harmful bacteria and great care must be given to the storage, handling and washing of raw vegetables in order to avoid contamination because of soil and soil dust.

*Insects and rodents*   Whatever steps are necessary must be taken to keep insects and rodents out of food premises. Most insects, flies especially, have hairy bodies which collect and distribute harmful bacteria. Flies land on animal faeces where they pick up large quantities on their bodies. They carry this to food items where they vomit and defecate on the food as they feed!

Rodents, both rats and mice, excrete organisms, such as *salmonella*, and contamination occurs from droppings, urine, hair and gnawing food containers etc. Mice use pipework, equipment etc., to gain entry to food premises and walk over surfaces. If this is suspected, the surfaces must be thoroughly sterilised and disinfected before use and entry points sealed. If you notice rodent droppings, these should be treated as a serious hazard and you should contact your *pest control officer* immediately. Always keep containers tightly lidded, as it is very difficult to tell the difference between currants and rodent droppings! Rodents usually run around the outside of rooms and therefore you will lessen any risk of contamination by not storing items around the walls of your storage areas.

*Animals and birds*   It is the hair and feathers on wild and domestic birds and animals which contain large amounts of harmful bacteria. This is very easily distributed if they are allowed into food premises. Even the cleanest of domestic pets have large quantities of harmful bacteria on their coats and when you stroke or pat them while they are in the food areas this bacteria is spread. Just allowing pets to wander around food premises means that they will rub against equipment and surfaces and so contaminate them.

*Dust*   There is always dust in the atmosphere and this contains many harmful bacteria. All foods should be kept well covered to make sure that dust particles cannot settle on the food and cause spoilage or contamination.

*Waste food and refuse*   This is a very important area to consider when dealing with contamination. Containers for refuse and waste food should be removed from the food area before they are anywhere near full. They should be made from materials which are easily disinfected and this should be done at the very least daily. Ideally there should be no facility for collecting waste food and refuse within the food area and chutes etc. should be installed to deal with removal of waste food and refuse.

Swill bins and refuse bins, by their very nature are breeding grounds for harmful bacteria and food-borne disease if they are not kept thoroughly cleaned and disinfected on a daily basis.

The storage area outside the premises (raised and tightly lidded containers) should also receive daily disinfection and cleaning, to discourage scavenging animals, birds and rodents.

Hands must be washed thoroughly after handling food waste and refuse.

Care must be taken to make sure that protective clothing does not become contaminated and bacteria transferred back into the food area.

One thing about bacteria which is most often misunderstood is that they *cannot* move by themselves; they have to be taken from one source to another.

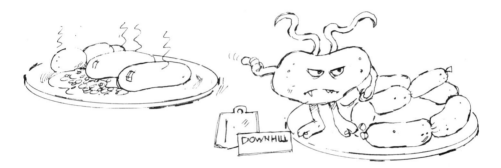

The movement of bacteria occurs by one or more of the following methods:

◆ Hands

◆ Cloths and equipment

◆ Hand-contact surfaces

◆ Food-contact surfaces

In most cases of food poisoning the bacteria have been transferred by *cross-contamination* where, for example, the food handler has transferred the bacteria to the food with his hands by not washing his hands after using the W.C. Another common cause is where raw foods have been prepared on a chopping board and then *high risk* foods placed immediately onto the board with little or no disinfection and so causing *cross-contamination*. Simply wiping the board with a soiled dish cloth is not sufficient to kill any harmful bacteria. It is more than likely that unless the cloth is kept in a solution of sterilant that the cloth contains more harmful bacteria than the board – in fact this is another perfect example of *cross-contamination*!

Chefs knives are also another common cause of *cross-contamination*. Unless they are sterilised after every process, it is highly likely that they will carry large numbers of harmful bacteria. Again, wiping with a soiled cloth simply increases the risk.

One area of the food room which does not get the attention it deserves is the *sink*. The food handler very often has dirty hands and turns the tap on, so passing debris and bacteria onto the tap. Once his hands are clean he then turns off the water – by touching the contaminated tap – and so the cycle of *cross-contamination* continues. At the end of a day's work, the taps, draining boards and outlets in the sinks will be absolutely *infested* with harmful bacteria which will have been spread all over the food area.

**Have a look around your food premises and see if you can see any areas which would allow *cross-contamination* to take place . . .**

Have you got covers on all internal swill and refuse containers?

Do you sterilise all wiping cloths, dish cloths, mops and buckets daily?

Are all raw vegetables stored well away from *high risk* foods?

Do you have raw and cooked foods stored in the same refrigerators/display cabinets?

How often do you disinfect the taps and outlets of your sinks?

Where do you keep the chemicals used for cleaning the food area?

> *Now complete the*
> *following questions at your own pace.*
> *When you have completed the questions check your*
> *answers by reading through Section 7 again.*
> *Mark your answers using the*
> *answer grid at the end*
> *of package*

**1**   Fill in the missing letters to complete the list of sources of bacteria which cause contamination.

   a)   T _ E   P _ R _ O _
   b)   R _ W   F _ O D _
   c)   _ N _ E _ T _
   d)   R _ D _ N _ S
   e)   A _ I _ A _ S
   f)   B _ R _ S
   g)   D _ S _
   h)   W _ S _ E   F _ O _ D
   i)   R _ F _ S _

**2**   'The moving of bacteria from raw foods to cooked foods without thought for correct food hygiene standards' would describe

   *a*   contamination
   *b*   cross-contamination
   *c*   food poisoning
   *d*   disinfection

**3**   **Bacterial contamination** is most likely to be caused by

   *a*   storage of cleaning materials in food areas
   *b*   lack of storage, washing and prep'n facilities
   *c*   doing maintenance work while preparing food
   *d*   use of unusual fruit, veg and plants in cookery

**4** **Chemical contamination** is most likely to be caused by

    *a* storage of cleaning materials in food areas
    *b* lack of storage, washing and prep'n facilities
    *c* doing maintenance work while preparing food
    *d* use of unusual fruit, veg and plants in cookery

**5** **Physical contamination** is most likely to be caused by

    *a* storage of cleaning materials in food areas
    *b* lack of storage, washing and prep'n facilities
    *c* doing maintenance work while preparing food
    *d* use of unusual fruit, veg and plants in cookery

**6** **Bacteria can move around the food preparation area by themselves** TRUE/FALSE

**7** It is a legal requirement that all cases of food poisoning are reported for investigation TRUE/FALSE

**8** Which of the following is most likely to cause cross-contamination?

    *a* ovens and stoves
    *b* small equipment
    *c* interiors of fridges and freezers
    *d* taps, fridge handles and oven control knobs

**9** Which of the following tasks in a food preparation area are most likely to cause cross contamination?

    *a* dicing raw meat
    *b* mincing livers for making pâté
    *c* opening and closing oven doors
    *d* moving immediately to sandwich preparation after trussing chickens

**10** You *must* wash your hands

    *a* before handling food waste and refuse
    *b* after handling food waste and refuse
    *c* before and after handling food waste and refuse

# SECTION EIGHT

# *Storage of food*

The correct storage of food is the key to any food business.
Satisfactory conditions of temperature control, cleanliness,
stock rotation and ventilation must be maintained to make
sure that good hygiene standards are achieved and controlled.

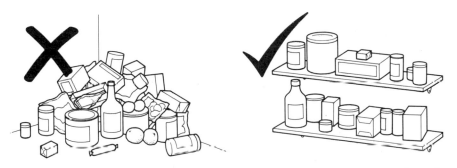

**Fig. 8.1**   *The correct storage of foods*

Lack of these basic requirements will result in food spoilage,
food unfit for human consumption, discoloration, staleness
and insect and rodent infestation. In order to maintain these
standards, adequate facilities in terms of storage space and
staff numbers must be provided. No matter how small a
business or how small an amount of food is to be stored there
should be separate areas set aside for each category of food
item purchased.

---

**Cleaning materials, chemicals, solvents etc., must be
stored completely separate from food stuffs so that no
contact is possible – in a different room from all food
storage and preparation.**

---

The main areas which need consideration when arranging storage facilities are: DRY-FOOD STORES, FRUIT AND VEGETABLE STORES, FROZEN FOOD STORES, REFRIGERATED STORES.

Obviously the amount of purchase you have will go a long way in deciding the amount of storage space you need. You should be careful that you do not store too much food simply because you have the storage room to accommodate it. Over stocking leads to food spoilage and encourages pest and insect infestation.

One commodity which is often overlooked when using or planning storage facilities is *adequate space* within the storage area to allow freedom of movement for stock controls and cleaning purposes. Where refrigerators are concerned you should always allow sufficient space between the fridges to allow movement of air. You should also pay particular attention to the amount of food you actually store in a refrigerator. Sufficient space between the foods stored is essential to maintain the circulation of cold air around the food stored. Overloading refrigerators is probably the most common cause of spoilage of perishable food items.

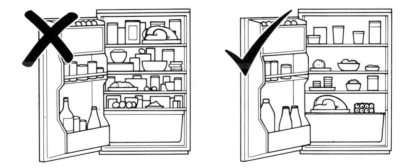

**Fig. 8.2** *The correct storage of refrigerated goods*

# Dry-food stores

This area is going to store dried and canned goods, cereals, flour, sugar, biscuits, tea, coffee and other non-perishable items.

◆ It must be dry, cool, well ventilated and lit, vermin proofed and kept clean and tidy

◆ No items what so ever should be stored directly on the floor and slatted stainless steel shelves or similar should be provided, starting at least 12″ from the floor

◆ Lidded, mobile bins should be provided for items such as flour and sugar to make sure that it is kept particularly dry and out of the reach of vermin and insects

◆ Shelving should not be too deep to reduce the possibility of stock being 'lost' at the back of shelves and so becoming spoiled and possibly contaminate other stock items

◆ Any spillages should be cleared up immediately and the floor, walls and corners of the area thoroughly cleaned on a regular basis

◆ To do this efficiently it is essential that space is left to allow movement of stock during your cleaning schedule

◆ All stock, especially canned goods, should be inspected for damage, rusting, infestation, out of date items etc., before storage

◆ Special attention should be given to identifying blown, dented and rusting cans

◆ Whenever new items are added to the stores the old items must be brought to the front of the shelves so that they are used first

◆ Strict stock rotation will reduce food spoilage and discourage pest infestation

## *Fruit and vegetable stores*

There are very few fruit and vegetables which will actually need refrigerated storage to keep them fresh. Fruit and vegetables should be purchased daily if possible, both to make sure of peak freshness and take advantage of price changes. A cool, well ventilated, dry area should be adequate for such storage with stainless steel, meshed shelving. Most fruit and vegetables are able to be stored in the containers you buy them in and transferring them to other containers only increases the risk of spoilage and contamination.

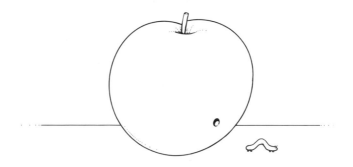

A very careful check of the condition of fruit and vegetables stored should be made daily as these commodities deteriorate very quickly and you can have a lot of food waste due to spoilage and contamination in a very short space of time.

> **Remember the old saying. . . . 'It only takes one bad apple'.**

# Frozen food stores

◆ Frozen foods need special attention. Many people think that because frozen food is safe from contamination and can be treated quite casually

◆ This is not so. In fact it is because the food is frozen that particular care has to be taken with it

◆ The area set aside for your freezer stores should be dry, well-ventilated and clean

◆ Make sure that the seals on freezer doors are working correctly and have regular maintenance checks made

◆ Make sure that your freezers are operating at the correct temperature to ensure that the internal temperature is sufficiently low enough to keep the foods frozen

> **Minus 18°C is the ideal operating temperature for freezers**

◆ Never store food above the *'Load line'* in freezers and check that new stock is placed beneath or behind old stock to ensure good stock rotation

◆ All frozen foods have a *shelf-life* (the length of time they are able to be stored, frozen, and still be suitable for human consumption). This shelf life should be checked regularly

◆ When accepting deliveries of frozen foods check that the food is at a suitable temperature and any found to be above minus 10°C should not be accepted

◆ Make absolutely sure that all frozen food deliveries are put straight into the freezers once they have been accepted from the suppliers

> **Never re-freeze foods which have thawed and not been used**

The frozen food you buy has been frozen commercially using *'Hi-tech'* methods which produce extremely small ice crystals within the food and reduce food spoilage and retain quality. When you use a 'domestic' freezer to re-freeze food the crystals which form are large and destroy the quality and texture of the food and increase the risk of spoilage.

Food which has thawed out will have risen in temperature and this rise in temperature allows bacteria on it to become more active and begin to grow and multiply.

If the food has simply been left open in the food area to thaw, it is likely that it will have been contaminated and again the bacteria transferred to it will have begun growing and multiplying. By re-freezing it you are simply storing food poisoning for a later date.

Foods which are stored in a freezer should be suitably wrapped. Just because bacteria are dormant at freezer temperatures does not mean that *cross-contamination* cannot take place.

Foods not suitably wrapped and protected can suffer from freezer burn which 'dries' up the surface of the food and results in food spoilage and loss of nutritional and presentation quality.

# The correct use of refrigerators

All perishable foods, especially *high risk foods* (dairy products, cooked meat, fish and poultry) should be stored in a refrigerator otherwise they can be contaminated by harmful bacteria.

Refrigeration at temperatures below 4°C retards most common food poisoning bacteria and they are unable to multiply at these temperatures – **but it does not kill the bacteria!** Spoilage of food by bacteria and mould is also reduced.

**Temperature control** is the single most significant factor in controlling bacteria growth and preventing food poisoning.

Most temperature control is done by keeping foods as cold as possible and so correct use of refrigerators is an essential part of hygiene training. Refrigerators should be sited in well ventilated areas where there is no heat source and out of direct sunlight.

Your refrigerator should be made of materials which are easily cleaned, with internal linings and shelves impervious and non-corroding. Door seals should be regularly checked and the whole unit serviced and maintained.

You should operate a frequent programme of defrosting and cleaning your refrigerator, at the very least, weekly, and you should avoid perfumed cleaning agents, using instead 1 table spoonful of Bicarbonate of Soda dissolved in 1 gallon of water.

## OPERATING TEMPERATURE

Your refrigerator should be set to operate at a temperature between **1°C and 4°C**. There should always be a thermometer placed in the warmest part of the refrigerator and readings checked and recorded **daily**.

Your refrigerator will only operate efficiently if you leave sufficient room around the foods stored in it, for the cold air to circulate.

By overloading the refrigerator you prevent the circulation

of the cold air and stop the unit working at its best temperature, and risk food spoilage and contamination.

◆ All foods stored in a refrigerator should be covered so that you can see immediately what is being stored and reduce the risk of cross contamination

◆ **Hot or even warm foods** should never be placed in a refrigerator

◆ How or warm foods placed into a refrigerator raise the temperature inside the fridge to levels which encourage bacterial growth and cause condensation which leads to cross contamination. It also makes the unit work harder to keep the best operating temperature and can result in burn out motors

◆ Never store food in opened tins or cans in a refrigerator as many canned goods contain acids which attack the can and cause contamination and food spoilage. (Fruit juices, tomato puree etc.).
   Part used cans of food should be transferred to plastic containers and covered before storing

◆ Avoid opening the doors of refrigerators more than is necessary and always close the doors immediately you have finished using the unit. The more the doors are left open the higher the internal temperature becomes and, as you now know, this leads to bacterial growth, contamination and food spoilage

Almost every home these days has a refrigerator and a freezer and if you look in most of the refrigerators you will see a combination of raw and cooked meats, dairy products etc.

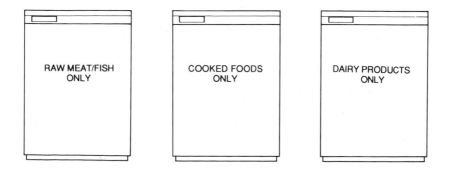

RAW MEAT/FISH ONLY

COOKED FOODS ONLY

DAIRY PRODUCTS ONLY

This combination is quite lethal and in the commercial world it is unacceptable. It is strongly recommended that the following rules should be followed for refrigerated storage of foods.

---

**A minimum of THREE refrigerators should be used to store products.**
**One for raw meats/fish products**
**One for cooked products**
**One for dairy products**

---

This use of three refrigerators reduces the risk of *cross-contamination* and allows a better system of stock rotation to be carried out.

Where only one fridge is used you must make absolutely sure that certain foods are stored on certain shelves within the fridge.

---

**Raw meats and fish on the bottom shelf.**
**Cooked foods on centre shelves.**
**Dairy products on top shelves.**

---

This prevents blood and liquid from thawing meats from dripping onto cooked and dairy foods (*high risk foods*) which may not be cooked or reheated before they are eaten.

Time must be taken making sure that all your older stock is used before new stock even in fridges and freezers.

During storage all your older stock should be constantly moved to the front of freezers, fridges etc., with the newer stock being placed behind.

Most food items now carry '**use by**' dates and these should be used to determine the amount of stock you purchase and which stock is used first. These date systems are an invaluable method of keeping efficient and hygienic stock rotation.

Manufacturers '**shelf-life**' stipulations should also be kept to as they have been calculated to make sure that the foods are protected from bacterial attack and spoilage if the dates are noted and acted upon.

Foods must be cooled down as quickly as possible after cooking if they are not going to be eaten immediately and stored in an efficient refrigerator (*within 1½ hours of cooking*) until required to stop the multiplication of harmful bacteria causing outbreaks of food poisoning.

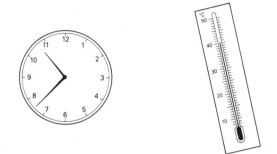

---

**Time and temperature controls are the critical factors in reducing harmful bacteria growth**

---

Foods should be kept out of the *danger zone* and the time between refrigeration and cooking, cooking and eating or cooking and refrigeration and refrigeration and serving, kept as short as possible.

Food does not have to look, smell, feel or even taste bad for it to be dangerous.

Food which is not to be eaten immediately after cooking must be kept at temperatures of above 65°C or below 5°C

*Now complete the
following questions at your own pace.
When you have completed the questions check your
answers by reading through Section 8 again.
Mark your answers using the
answer grid at the end
of package*

**1**    The ideal operating temperature for a freezer is

    *a*  18°C
    *b*  −18°C
    *c*  37°C
    *d*  −37°C

**2**    The ideal operating temperature for a refrigerator is

    *a*  1°C–4°C
    *b*  5°C–65°C
    *c*  18°C
    *d*  37°C

**3**    A refrigerator operates best when it is packed with food.    TRUE/FALSE

**4**    What would be the best type of shelving to use in a dry stores?

    *a*  slatted wooden shelving
    *b*  solid wooden shelving
    *c*  slatted stainless steel shelving
    *d*  solid stainless steel shelving

**5**    It is important that old stock is used before new stock. What is the term which describes this procedure?

    _____ _____

**6**   All frozen foods are completely safe from contamination.   TRUE/FALSE

**7**   It is perfectly acceptable to place warm foods in a refrigarator to cool them down quickly.                                      TRUE/FALSE

**8**   Constantly opening and closing refrigerator doors increases the risk of bacteria multiplication.                              TRUE/FALSE

**9**   Which of the following statements is correct?

   *a*   Cooking food makes it safe from contamination
   *b*   Contaminated food looks, smells, feels and tastes normal
   *c*   Frozen chickens are best thawed under warm running water
   *d*   The operating temperature of a fridge is − 18°C

**10**  Ideally you should have three fridges for the storage of foods. What should be stored in each?

   *a*   _____

   *b*   _____

   *c*   _____

**11**  Food which has been cooked and required to be served cold must be cooled down within

   *a*   24 hours
   *b*   12 hours
   *c*   4 hours
   *d*   1½ hours

**12**  Refrigeration and freezing kills harmful bacteria.            TRUE/FALSE

**13**  Food which is not to be eaten immediately after cooking must be kept at temperatures of

   *a*   above 65°C or below 5°C
   *b*   above 50°C or below 5°C
   *c*   above 37°C or below 5°C
   *d*   above 18°C or below 5°C

**14**  There is no need to operate stock rotation for foods stored in fridges or freezers.                                           TRUE/FALSE

**15**  Where there is only one fridge in the kitchen all raw meat and poultry
should be stored on the top shelf.                TRUE/FALSE

**16**  Opened cans of food should never be stored in a fridge.    TRUE/FALSE

**17**  It is always safest to cover foods stored in a fridge.        TRUE/FALSE

**18**  Frozen food can safely be stored in a frozen condition
indefinitely.                                      TRUE/FALSE

# SECTION NINE

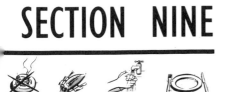

# *Thawing frozen foods*

With the modern techniques available today it is quite possible to cook many items straight from the freezer, without thawing. Many items in fact must not be thawed, due to the way in which they have been manufactured. Small pieces of meat and poultry, pre-cooked and re-formed items of fish, meat and poultry come under this heading. However, large joints of meat and *all* frozen, whole birds *must* be completely thawed before cooking.

## *Poultry*

All frozen foods, especially poultry, must be thawed out in a refrigerator and *never* by placing under warm running water.

Poultry is a notorious source of salmonella bacteria and great care must be taken when thawing to reduce the risk of cross contamination from the thawing liquid which can contaminate chopping boards, work surfaces, equipment, knives and clothing.

By thawing under running warm water the surface of the poultry thaws far quicker than the inside of the bird and allows bacteria the ideal conditions of warmth and moisture which they need to multiply and grow. It is very probable that the centre of the bird is not thoroughly thawed out when the flesh of the bird is quite thawed and this can result in poultry being placed in the oven when it is only partially thawed.

The sink, waste outlet and taps of the sink are also heavily contaminated with the thawing liquid (freezer drip) and are usually the areas which do not receive adequate disinfection when the poultry is removed for cooking. The risk of *cross-*

*contamination* from the sink and taps is extremely great.

> **Cooked foods which are cooling before being refrigerated must never be in the same area as thawing meat or poultry.**
>
> **The ideal way to make sure that frozen foods are completely thawed is to use a digital probe thermometer to check the temperature of the centre of the thawing food.**

## *RULES FOR HANDLING FROZEN POULTRY*

Frozen poultry of any kind should be handled with great care. Poultry is one of the most common causes of food poisoning and cannot be given enough care during storage, preparation, cooking and serving.

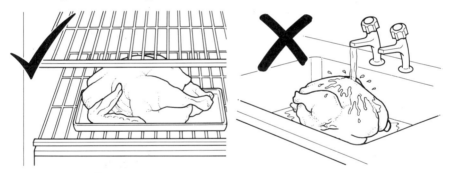

◆ Always store frozen poultry separately from other frozen foods (at the very least in separate freezer baskets/divisions in the freezer) – ideally in a separate freezer

◆ Thaw poultry completely in a refrigerator. Thawing is only complete when the body is pliable, the legs flexible and the body cavity *100% free of ice crystals*

◆ Once thawed, poultry should be cooked immediately or kept in a refrigerator and cooked within 24 hours

◆ Always remove the giblets, prior to cooking. *Never* cook poultry with the giblets inside the bird

◆ If the poultry is to be stuffed then this should be done from the neck end and *never by filling the body cavity*. Ideally the stuffing should be cooked separately. The body cavity is very moist and when it is filled with stuffing, which contains breadcrumbs, the moisture is absorbed into the stuffing.

The stuffing forms a very dense mass and the heat of the oven is unlikely to penetrate to the centre of the stuffing before the bird itself is cooked. This leaves the stuffing only partially cooked and in the ideal conditions for bacteria to grow and multiply.

Unless the poultry is served immediately this bacterial growth continues unchecked and by the time the poultry is served it is literally infested with food poisoning bacteria and an outbreak of poisoning is virtually guaranteed

◆ All utensils, work surfaces, equipment and sink outlets and taps used to prepare raw meat and poultry must be thoroughly disinfected after use and never used to prepare cooked foods without such cleaning and disinfection

◆ Once cooked, poultry should be eaten straight away. If it is to be served cold then it must be cooled down rapidly (within $1\frac{1}{2}$ hours), ideally through a blast chiller and stored in a refrigerator until required which should be within 12 hours of cooking

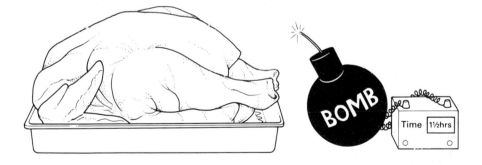

---

**All meats, including poultry, should be brought to a temperature at which they can be refrigerated within $1\frac{1}{2}$ hours after cooking if not served straight away.**

---

◆ Avoid handling cooked poultry as much as possible to reduce the risk of cross-contamination

*Now complete the
following questions at your own pace.
When you have completed the questions check your
answers by reading through Section 9 again.
Mark your answers using the
answer grid at the end
of package*

**1**  Foods which have been cooked and are not to be served hot must be cooled down and refrigerated within

   *a*  24 hours
   *b*  12 hours
   *c*  3 hours
   *d*  1½ hours.

**2**  Ideally where should this cooling process be carried out?

   *a*  in a refrigerator
   *b*  in a cool room
   *c*  in a blast chiller
   *d*  in the kitchen overnight

**3**  Frozen foods can be stored in a freezer for

   *a*  1 month
   *b*  2 months
   *c*  3 months
   *d*  according to instruction on the packet.

**4**  Frozen foods which are delivered at a temperature of above −10°C should be

   *a*  placed immediately in the freezer
   *b*  used straight away
   *c*  returned to supplier
   *d*  allowed to thaw out completely and stored in fridge

**5** It is acceptable to re-freeze unopened packets of thawed
foods. TRUE/FALSE

**6** You only have one fridge in the kitchen. Where, in the fridge, should you
place a joint of fresh beef?

*a* on the top shelf
*b* above any dairy products stored in fridge
*c* in the centre of the fridge
*d* on a tray at the bottom of the fridge

**7** All equipment, utensils and work surfaces should be disinfected after
thawing frozen poultry. TRUE/FALSE

**8** How should stuffing for poultry be cooked in order to ensure thorough
cooking and minimise bacterial growth?

*a* in the body cavity of the bird
*b* separately from the bird
*c* in the neck end of the bird

# SECTION TEN

# *Design of food premises*

## *Essential requirements*

When ever food premises are built, adapted or planned it is very often only the food preparation or service areas which are given any degree of thought or consideration. To make sure that a high standard of working hygiene is achieved the actual *location* of the premises must be considered.

While it may seem obvious, you need to think about:

◆ **Suitable electricity supply**. You will need to make sure that you have the necessary supply for single and three phase equipment

◆ **Suitable gas supply**. You will need to make sure that you can actually have a gas supply or whether you would consider Calor Gas etc.

◆ **Suitable water supply**. You will need to make absolutely sure that a supply of treated water is available and in the quantities you will require

◆ **Suitable sewage system**. You will need to make sure that the premises have a suitable sewage system

◆ **Suitable delivery access**. You will need to make sure that there is suitable access for delivery vehicles etc.

◆ **Suitable refuse disposal service**. You will need to make sure that there is a suitable refuse disposal service or arrange a private contract for the removal of refuse from the premises

Once these things have been considered and arranged then you must look at the actual construction and design of the premises themselves.

There are a lot of different things which have to be thought of and considered when planning or designing food premises so that they can operate in an easy hygienic and safe way.

◆ There must be completely separate areas within the premises which are identified for specific tasks. For example, you do not want to have the washing up area or vegetable preparation areas next to, or part of the cooking areas. There are certain food preparation sections which must be completely separate – preparation of cooked foods and preparation of raw foods and meats

  Great thought must be given so that the whole operation 'flows' through the premises and there is not a continuous 'criss-crossing' which will lead to a high risk of cross contamination

◆ Adequate refrigeration, cooking, cooling and chilling and storage areas should be available to make sure that the food does not become contaminated

◆ Adequate provision for *personal hygiene standards* must be made.

  Wash hand basins, with suitable supplies of hot and cold water, nail brushes and soap must be provided next to W.C.'s. There must be suitable provision of washing facilities for equipment to allow cleaning and disinfection to take place.

  Separate facilities must be made for the washing of food stuffs and these must never be used for washing equipment, hands etc.

  Suitable supplies of hot and cold water must be made to the premises

◆ The premises should be constructed to allow thorough cleaning and disinfection to take place with the minimum of effort

◆ Suitable arrangements to stop rodents and insects gaining access to the premises should be made

◆ Staff facilities, such as locker rooms, rest rooms etc., should be provided

◆ Satisfactory ventilation, air conditioning and lighting must be provided to allow efficient temperature controls and working conditions to be achieved

# *Internal design principles*

There are certain specific design principles which have to be considered when deciding the internal details of the premises.

## *CEILINGS*

Ceilings should be smooth, light coloured, fire resistant, durable and *coved* at all wall joints. They should be decorated so that they are easily cleaned.

\* **Coving – coving is when the joints of walls and ceilings** *or* walls and floors are finished off in a curve rather than a right angle.

This prevents a build up of dirt, dust and debris forming at these joints, which contain harmful bacteria, and makes efficient cleaning a lot easier.

RIGHT ANGLED JOINT        COVED JOINT

## *WINDOWS*

Where ever possible windows should be on north facing walls to reduce glare and solar heat build-up. All windows should be fitted with fly screens which are easily cleaned.

Window sills should be made so that they are sloping away from the window or be very shallow to allow easier cleaning and not able to be used as 'storage areas' for foods or plants etc.

## *WALLS*

Walls should be smooth, light coloured, durable, impervious (not absorbent), and capable of being *thoroughly* and easily cleaned. In the normal course of a days work the walls will become spotted with food debris etc. and must be able to withstand heat, impact and thorough disinfection.

Internal walls should be solid as cavity walls can easily harbour pests and rodents.

Where tiles are fitted to the walls they should be flush to the wall, with no gaps beneath as this is where insects etc., can live and breed.

(A much better material for walls, rather than tiles, is *polypropylene* panels with welded seams. This method provides a thoroughly hygienic finish to all walls etc. and is very much easier to keep hygienic – think of trying to clean dirty grouting!)

## FLOOR SURFACES

The most important thing to consider with *floors* is that they are able to be easily cleaned and that they are as *non-slip* as possible. Floors will take a lot of punishment both while working and when being cleaned and so they must be able to withstand impact, very hot liquids and cleaning chemicals.

If at all possible floors should be laid with sufficient slope, leading to gullies, to allow spilt and cleaning liquids to be disposed of easily and safely without the necessity for mops and buckets.

Mops and buckets are notorious for not being kept in a hygienic condition and, unfortunately are often 'alive' with harmful bacteria, which is simply spread around food areas when floors are 'cleaned'.

If gullies are fitted in the floors they can be thoroughly hosed down and the water allowed to drain into these gullies without the need for mops etc.

## WOODEN FINISHES

Ideally there should be no wooden finishes at all in food areas. If it is necessary, for example, window frames etc., then these must be made of well-seasoned hardwood, treated with primer and have at least three coats of polyurethane paint.

## EQUIPMENT

All plant equipment within a food area should be sited at least 12" from the outer walls to allow for adequate and thorough cleaning to take place easily. if this is not possible then the equipment should be fitted on rollers to allow easy movement for regular cleaning to take place.

> **Throughout the whole of the food premises the emphasis must be on the ease of thorough cleaning and all surfaces and equipment must be able to be cleaned with the minimum of effort.**

*Now complete
the following questions at your own pace.
When you have completed the questions check your
answers by reading through Section 10 again.
Mark your answers using the
answer grid at the end
of package*

**1**   It is a legal requirement that food premises must have a suitable supply of hot and cold water.                              TRUE/FALSE

**2**   In order to reduce the possibility of cross-contamination there should be separate areas within the food premises for the preparation of raw and cooked foods.                              TRUE/FALSE

**3**   What facilities must be provided at wash hand basins in food premises?

   *a*   hot and cold water
   *b*   nailbrush and soap
   *c*   system for drying your hands
   *d*   all of these facilities.

**4**   Wash hand basins with necessary facilities *must* be provided immediately
      adjacent to WC's.                                                          TRUE/FALSE

**5**   Make a simple diagram, below, of what you understand by a *coved joint*.

**6**   The walls in food preparation areas must be able to be cleaned
      easily.                                                                    TRUE/FALSE

**7**   Heavy equipment in a food premises must be able to be moved to allow
      ease of cleaning.                                                          TRUE/FALSE

**8**   The lack of adequate refrigeration, cooking, cooling and storage areas
      within a food premises will contribute to contamination of
      food.                                                                      TRUE/FALSE

# SECTION ELEVEN

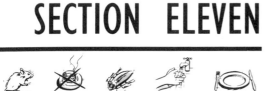

# *Equipment used in food premises*

All equipment, surfaces, hand tools etc., which are bought for use in the food industry should be given special consideration regarding hygiene. Not only should the equipment etc., do the job it was bought for but it must also be able to be cleaned and disinfected easily. All equipment, large or small, should be able to be thoroughly sterilised and disinfected with the minimum effort or trouble.

If any piece of equipment is difficult to clean, sterilise or disinfect then it is more than likely that this *essential* job will not be done properly. This will mean that there will be a gradual build up of debris and harmful bacteria and so increase the risk of cross-contamination throughout the food area.

The equipment can be something as simple as a potato masher or sieve, which has little nooks and crannies which are difficult to get clean. Staff may not have the time or patience to clean them properly and eventually they become infested with harmful bacteria.

## *DURABILITY*

Equipment should be bought which will last and not fall to pieces or become damaged easily. Replacement of equipment is expensive and very often damaged equipment is kept in use even when it is a danger to the food it is being used to prepare or serve. For example, cups, plates etc., which are chipped and cracked harbour thousands, if not millions, of harmful bacteria and are a grave risk to health. **Any chipped, cracked or damaged crockery etc., should be thrown out immediately**.

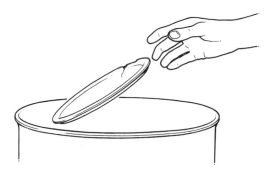

## MATERIALS USED IN MANUFACTURE

You should consider very carefully what materials are used to actually make the equipment you are buying. If the material is a metal then you should make sure that it is completely rust proof and that it will stand up to the impacts, knocks and bangs it is likely to get when it is used.

Plastics etc., should be looked at very carefully as some can be liable to melt at fairly low temperatures and may become dissolved into foods. Others are very brittle and if they chip or are dropped, pieces may land in foods and cause physical contamination.

**Wood should not be used for any equipment whatsoever.** Wood is very absorbent and difficult to keep sterilised and in normal use gets marked, pitted and cracked. This leads to a build up of harmful bacteria which can very quickly cause food poisoning and cross-contamination.

## WORK BENCHES AND SURFACES

Should be made of stainless steel as this is durable and able to be sterilised very easily.

## CHOPPING BOARDS

Should be made of polyurethane or other suitable material which is able to withstand regualr sterilisation. Chopping boards should get special attention when they are purchased and it is chopping boards which contribute to a large percentage of cases of cross-contamination.

Specific boards should be used for specific jobs in the food area and it is now possible to buy *coloured* polyurethane chopping boards so that a different coloured board can be used for different tasks.

The different tasks which would need separate boards would be:

◆ Preparation of raw meat and chicken

◆ Preparation of raw fish

◆ Preparation of cooked foods

◆ Preparation of raw vegetables

◆ Preparation of dairy products

It is also possible to buy knives with matching colour-coded handles to the boards and greatly help in reducing the risk of cross-contamination.

## SHELVING

Should be metal and coated in an easily cleanable material and preferably be slatted rather than solid. Where shelves are placed around walls they should be sited at least 2–3″ away from the wall so that the shelf and the wall behind can be thoroughly cleaned and disinfected easily.

## DRAWERS

Should not be used in food premises. They are difficult to clean and are the obvious place for the build up of dirt, dust and debris, and therefore bacteria.

*Where do you 'hide' equipment?*    If there are drawers available you will find that they are just the 'hiding place' needed by inexperienced or careless staff for that equipment which isn't as clean as it should be or difficult to clean!

All equipment should be cleaned and sterilised immediately after use and a regular system of cleaning operated for equipment and utensils which are not used very often. Every piece of equipment which is not used on a regular basis should be cleaned and sterilised weekly at the very least. Equipment which is not used regularly can become the home for rodents and pests unless it gets frequent attention.

> **Any equipment which is broken should be removed from the food area until it is repaired or replaced.**

*Now complete
the following questions at your own pace.
When you have completed the questions check your
answers by reading through Section 11 again.
Mark your answers using the
answer grid at the end
of package*

**I** The prime hygiene consideration when buying equipment for use within food premises is that it should be able to be cleaned and disinfected easily.      TRUE/FALSE

**2** Providing that chipped and cracked equipment is disinfected regularly there is no danger of contamination.      TRUE/FALSE

**3** Both large and small equipment in food premises should be cleaned and disinfected

   *a*  only after use
   *b*  when necessary
   *c*  on a regular basis whether used or not
   *d*  monthly.

**4**   What is the main reason why wooden chopping boards are not suitable for use in food premises?

   *a*  they are very heay to carry
   *b*  they are absorbent and harbour bacteria
   *c*  they are expensive to buy
   *d*  they can splinter and injure staff.

**5**   Stainless steel work benches are ideal in food premises because

   *a*  they rarely need replacing
   *b*  they are very stable and do not move easily
   *c*  they are easily disinfected
   *d*  they provide a cold surface for cold preparation

**6**   Small equipment should be stored where it is always visible.                                    TRUE/FALSE

# SECTION TWELVE

# *Storage and disposal of waste*

Just look at the title of this section for a second. . . .

No-one actually stores waste food etc., surely? Disposal of waste, certainly, but *storage*!

Then ask yourself this question . . . 'Do you always take waste items, immediately to waste containers *outside* the food premises?'

Your answer must be **NO**.

Therefore you store it!

The storage and disposal of waste is not given very much consideration or importance when dealing with food preparation and production. Yet cross-contamination, food poisoning and especially food-borne diseases are quite often the result of badly stored waste materials from food premises.

Waste material must be given the same consideration as you would give to preparing a gourmet banquet, or creating a masterpiece gateau etc. There is far less chance of causing illness from these two exercises than there is from badly stored waste materials.

Before we continue with this section just look around the areas where the waste materials are stored and disposed of in the establishments where you work and see if they are clean, tidy and free from spillages.

The containers which are used for the storage of waste materials should be made of material which is easily sterilised and disinfected and they should not be so large that collection or emptying them need not take place for a number of days.

Ideally, containers used inside the premises, should be plastic and be small enough to require emptying at least three times every working day.

Containers for storing waste outside the premises must be sited on a raised platform to discourage scavenging by animals, rodents and birds.

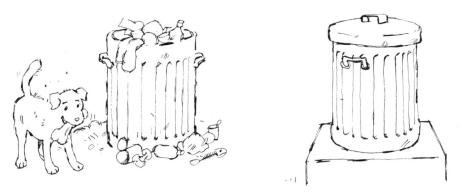

---

**Internal and external use containers must be fitted with secure lids**

---

All containers used for storage of waste must be emptied regularly and especially before they become too full. It is more hygienic to have these containers lined with polythene sacks which can be tied securely once they are *half full* and again, this reduces the risk of scavenging or the contents being spilt and scattered.

Spillages from waste containers cause many incidents of food related illness as food handlers are inclined simply to pick up spillages and return them to the containers without then thoroughly washing their hands or considering that bacteria could have been transferred onto their clothing and so spread harmful bacteria throughout the food areas.

---

**Hands must always be washed after handling waste and refuse**

---

The storage of returnable containers, such as bread trays, crates etc., should also be given a high priority and kept in a clean, dry area, preferably under cover (as protection from soiling by animals, rodents and birds) until they are collected by suppliers. You should also inspect the containers which your goods are delivered in to make sure that they are as clean as possible – especially milk crates and other dairy product containers.

*Now complete
the following questions at your own pace.
When you have completed the questions check your
answers by reading through Section 12 again.
Mark your answers using the
answer grid at the end
of package*

1  What main consideration should be given to containers used for storing waste and refuse?

   *a*  light to handle
   *b*  large enough to take all refuse for a days work
   *c*  brightly coloured for identification
   *d*  lidded and easily disinfected.

2  Many cases of food related illnesses are caused by incorrect handling of food waste and refuse.                    TRUE/FALSE

3  Refuse containers sited outside the building should be raised off the ground and securely lidded to prevent

   *a*  bad smells and odours
   *b*  scavenging by birds, animals and rodents
   *c*  spillages

4  Your hands must be washed thoroughly AFTER handling waste and refuse.                    TRUE/FALSE

**5**   Returnable containers which food is delivered in can safely be stored
      outside until collected.                                    TRUE/FALSE

**6**   There is no risk of contamination and possible food poisoning from
      returnable food containers.                                 TRUE/FALSE

# SECTION THIRTEEN

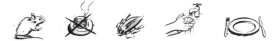

# Cleaning food premises

Before we start this important section there are three words which have been used already in the training package but which we need to understand a little more.

**DETERGENT     DISINFECTANT     SANITISER**

Go back to pages 1–2 to refresh your memory of these definitions.

Another word which we should explain at this stage is cleaning.

*Cleaning* is the removal of food debris, grease or dirt.

## The cleaning process

*Everyone knows how to clean, don't they? Of course they do, they have done it a thousand times!*

You must have cleaned up more times than you can remember. You will have cleaned floors, benches, cupboards, dishes, equipment, etc.

*So how did you do it then?*

Spend a couple of minutes thinking about any cleaning job you have done and try and break it down into invidivual stages. Just to give you a bit of help, you should be able to find **six** stages within any cleaning operation.

*How have you got on then?*

O.K. here are the six basic stages in any cleaning operation.

◆ Pre-clean – this is the removal of dirt, debris, soil etc. by wiping, sweeping, scraping or pre-rinsing

Main clean – this is the loosening of the surface grease, dirt etc. by using a detergent

 Rinse – this is the removal of all dirt, debris etc. AND the removal of the detergent used in the main clean

 Disinfection – this is the destroying of bacteria using a disinfectant (non-perfumed, of course), steam or water at 82°C and above

 Final rinse – this is the removal of traces of disinfectant

 Drying – this is the drying of the articles using clean cloths or preferably by *air drying* which is by letting the articles dry in the air without using any cloths etc.

If a sanitiser is used then stages 2–4 are combined.

## *Effective cleaning*

Now that you know the six basic stages in any cleaning operation, can you in all honesty say that you *always* go through every one of the six stages when ever you clean anything?

Any cleaning programme, to be beneficial and efficient, must be planned: the frequency of the cleaning; the degree of cleaning; the chemicals and amount of chemicals to be used; the staff responsible for the cleaning operation decided, and the supervision for the cleaning operation determined.

Once the complete programme has been finalised it must be carried out very strictly. It is no use missing part of it out, because 'there isn't time to-day', or because 'there isn't any of that pink powder left'!

One of the most important and easy ways of making sure that you don't have to undertake mammoth cleaning operations everyday is to *train staff* to *clean as they go* – if this can be done then a great deal of cleaning operation is carried out during the working day, with very little effort and trouble.

Extreme care must be taken when dealing with chemicals for cleaning processes and **under no circumstances** should open food be exposed to the risk of contamination during cleaning operations.

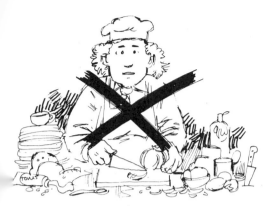 

## WHAT IS CLEANING?

We have already decided that cleaning means *the removal of food debris, grease or dirt*.

Once you have cleaned efficiently and thoroughly you must then *disinfect* in order to destroy the harmful bacteria which can remain on the articles. The most efficient way of doing this is by using hot water (82°C), steam and diluted bleaches – which are the most common disinfectants.

Disinfectant solutions should be made up as required as stale disinfectant solutions actually attract bacteria growth.

Leaving mops soaking in disinfectant solution overnight is not such a good idea!

## WHAT NEEDS DISINFECTION?

◆ All hand-contact surfaces – knives, small equipment, door handles and all hand tools etc. and everything your hands touch during your working day. Especially surfaces in washrooms and W.C.'s

◆ All food-contact surfaces – everything which the food touches during its storage, preparation, cooking and serving

◆ All equipment – every piece of equipment which is used in the premises must be disinfected on a regular basis and not only after use

◆ Your hands – the food handler must make sure that his hands are disinfected thoroughly at all times during the working day. Washing is not sufficient

## WHY DO WE CLEAN?

Cleaning is done for the following reasons:

To promote a favourable and acceptable image to customers and staff

 To remove material on which bacteria can grow and multiply and which might cause contamination, food poisoning or food-borne disease

◆ To ensure a safe and hygienic working environment

◆ To allow disinfection of equipment and surfaces

◆ To remove materials which could encourage pest and insect infestation

◆ To reduce the risk of physical contamination

*Washing*
Washing is a form of cleaning and the washing of equipment, crockery etc., should be given special attention.

It is more than likely that most small equipment, crockery, glassware, cutlery etc., is washed through dishwashing machines, where all the food handler has to do is to switch on the pre-set controls and load and unload the machine. The machine will have been set to go through the six basic stages of the cleaning operation automatically and have been filled with the necessary detergent, disinfectant and rinsing chemicals.

(The food handler normally has to do the *pre-clean* by hand unless a powerful spray is fitted to the machine for this purpose).

Regular checks will ensure that water temperatures and chemicals used in dishwashing machines are operating correctly.

> **\* Don't forget that mops and brushes should also be washed, disinfected and left to dry after use!**

There are often, times during the day, where using a dishwashing machine for washing up is neither convenient or possible. In these cases it is necessary to wash up by hand in sinks and then the following system is recommended:

*Double sink washing*
◆ Remove heavy or loose debris by scraping into a lidded refuse container, and rinsing the article in cold water

◆ Place the articles into the first sink, containing detergent and water at a temperature of *50°C–60°C, use a brush or cloth to remove dirt and grease. Change the water as often as it gets cool or dirty

◆ Place the articles into the second sink to rinse off traces of the detergent and leave for 30 seconds in water at *82°C to achieve disinfection

* 50°C–60°C – the water for washing the dishes etc., should be at a temperature of between 50°C–60°C (certainly no hotter) so that it assists the detergent in removing debris. If the water were any hotter there is a good chance that it would actually 'bake or cook' the debris on to the article.

* 82°C – the water for rinsing the articles should be at least 82°C so that it is capable of killing off all harmful bacteria which may still be on them and so achieve effective disinfection.

*Now complete
the following questions at your own pace.
When you have completed the questions check your
answers by reading through Section 13 again.
Mark your answers using the
answer grid at the end
of package*

| A chemical used to remove grease, dirt and food debris is a

   *a* disinfectant
   *b* sterilant
   *c* detergent
   *d* bactericide

**2** A disinfectant is used to

   *a*  kill all harmful bacteria
   *b*  reduce harmful bacteria to a safe level
   *c*  help remove grease and food debris
   *d*  make dishes and crockery sparkle after washing

**3** The ideal temperature of water for washing food preparation equipment is

   *a*  82–85°C
   *b*  30–37°C
   *c*  50–60°C
   *d*   5–65°C

**4** The ideal temperature of water for disinfecting food preparation equipment is

   *a*  82–85°C
   *b*  30–37°C
   *c*  50–60°C
   *d*   5–65°C

**5** How often should the water for washing dishes and equipment be changed when using the double sink method

   *a*  once
   *b*  twice
   *c*  when it gets cool
   *d*  when it gets cool or dirty

**6** What would be most important when cleaning floors in food preparation areas?

   *a*  always leave floors wet
   *b*  always use a caustic solution
   *c*  remove all dirt and debris using hot water and detergent before disinfecting
   *d*  clean floors daily

**7**   Disinfectants should be

    *a*  made as strong as possible
    *b*  made up each time they are needed
    *c*  stored in the food preparation area
    *d*  used instead of detergent

# SECTION FOURTEEN

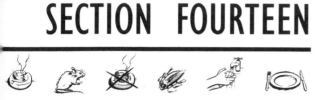

# *Pest control*

This section of the training package will deal with *food pests*.

A *food pest* is an animal which lives either in or on food and causes destruction, contamination or is troublesome.

The common pests you are likely to find on food premises are:

**Rodents**, such as rats and mice.

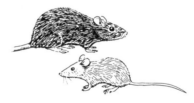

**Insects**, such as flies, cockroaches, silverfish, ants and stored product insects.

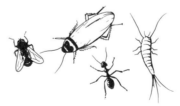

**Birds**, such as sparrows and wild pigeons.

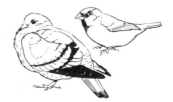

All the above food pests are likely to cause damage, contaminate food or generally be a nuisance if they are allowed to live on food premises.

It is important that you are always on the look out for signs which can tell you that there are food pests on food premises. These would include:

◆ Live or dead bodies, including larvae or pupae in and around the food premises

◆ Rodents droppings

◆ Damage to sacks, packages, boxes etc. caused by rodents gnawing and clawing actions

◆ Spillages near sacks of food etc., which would show that pests had damaged them

◆ Rodent smears around pipework

A careful watch for any of these tell-tale signs will allow you to take quick action to get rid of the food pests.

## Why do we need to control food pests?

Whenever there are pests on food premises there is a grave risk of contamination, food spoilage, food poisoning and food-borne disease as none of the pests have particularly hygienic habits.

The reasons for controlling pests are, to prevent the spread of disease, to prevent damage, to prevent food wastage and *to comply with the law.*

Just like all other living things, pests need food, shelter and security in order to survive. If you deny them these basic requirements then they are not going to stay or even come onto food premises.

Food premises should be planned and operated so that pests do not find the conditions they need to survive and so cause infestation.

The two main ways therefore, of controlling food pests are by *denying them access to the premises* and *denying them food and shelter.*

# *How can you control pests?*

Before we look at how to control pests, we had better think about where the most likely places to find pests on food premises would be.

Pests like shelter and warmth and they don't like being disturbed so the places to keep a special watch are store rooms which contain items which are not used very frequently.

◆ Stores for cleaning equipment such as brushes, mops, buckets

◆ Stores for paper goods, bags, wrapping paper, boxes etc.

◆ Stores for equipment which is waiting to be repaired

Pests do not necessarily require what we call *food* to live. For example, rodents are quite happy eating *soap*!

Anywhere which is not kept clean and tidy regularly:

◆ Old out buildings, sheds, garages, etc.

◆ Sheds where gardening equipment is stored

◆ Those awkward corners of old food premises which have been used to 'dump' all the bits and pieces which nobody has time to get rid of!

One obvious area is the waste and swill area, especially if it is not kept disinfected and clean on a regular basis. There is also a great risk of attracting pests to food premises if there is any amount of untended shrubbery etc., very close to the premises.

It is as important to 'look around' food premises to see if there is anything which would be an attraction for pests – rodents, insects or birds.

# DENY PESTS ACCESS TO PREMISES

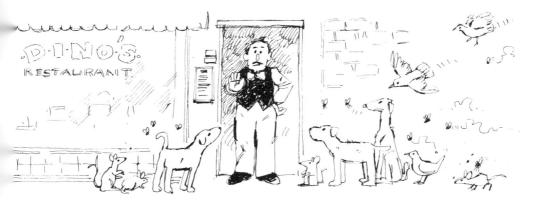

Operate thorough, systematic cleaning, disinfection and tidying programmes throughout the premises and the immediate surrounding area.

◆ Install cleanable mesh at all windows

◆ Always carry out regular maintenance inspections and make sure that every job fault found is dealt with immediately

> **Prevention is better than cure!**

◆ Install ultra violet insect killers

◆ Box in pipework in and around the premises and make 100% sure that where pipes etc., enter the buildings that these are completely sealed. A mouse can squeeze through a space the size of a hole made by poking a pencil through a sheet of paper!

◆ Spend time and thought when designing or altering premises to proofing them against pests.

◆ Make sure that doors fit securely and there are no gaps for pests to gain entry. Fit strong metal 'kick plates' to all outer doors ﹘ rats can gnaw through fairly thick metal if they are determined to get into premises!

# DENY PESTS FOOD AND SHELTER

Make sure that the premises and refuse areas are *always* kept clean, tidy and thoroughly disinfected.

◆ Always have spillages removed as soon as they happen

◆ Always store food off the floor (12" from ground) and away from walls to allow easy and regular inspections to take place. (Rodents prefer to keep to the outer edges of rooms)

◆ Always store food in lidded containers (metal preferably) and see that lids are replaced immediately after use

◆ Make sure that the surrounding areas of the food premises are kept in good repair and are regularly tidied

◆ Always check deliveries to the premises to make sure that there are no pests etc. being brought into the premises with deliveries. As with most things it is quite simply a system of 'good housekeeping' which goes a long way to making sure that food pests are not encouraged onto food premises

It is much better if you can actually stop food pests getting into food premises but if it does happen you are going to have to use physical or chemical means of getting rid of them.

If you do get infestation the best course of action is to call in your local pest control officer immediately who can take specialist action to rid the premises which may mean a number of visits before the problem is solved.

*Now complete
the following questions at your own pace.
When you have completed the questions check your
answers by reading through Section 14 again.
Mark your answers using the
answer grid at the end
of package*

**I** The *main* reason why food pests must be controlled is that they

    *a* add to the cleaning duties
    *b* spread disease
    *c* are unpleasant to staff and customers
    *d* can spoil food

**2** Rats and mice will not be attracted to your premises if you

    *a* keep a cat
    *b* lay traps and poison
    *c* keep all doors closed
    *d* keep everything clean and disinfected

**3** Flies can be best controlled in food preparation areas by

    *a* using fly papers
    *b* using fly sprays
    *c* using ultra violet insect killer
    *d* keeping all windows closed

**4** Food pests are

    *a* rats and mice
    *b* flies and cockroaches
    *c* cats, dogs and birds
    *d* all of these

**5** If you notice signs of rats and mice on food premises you should

    *a* clean and disinfect the area
    *b* lay traps
    *c* lay poison
    *d* contact your local pest control officer

**6** Which of the following statements is correct?

    *a* pests in the kitchen are not a danger if all food is kept covered and stored at least 12″ off the ground
    *b* domestic pets can be allowed in the food preparation area when the area is closed
    *c* pests and domestic pets must not be allowed in food preparation areas
    *d* domestic pets are no danger in food preparation areas.

**7** The two main ways of controlling food pests are to
        **Deny them _OO_ and ___LT_R**

# SECTION FIFTEEN

# The law relating to food and food hygiene

As with any laws, those concerning food and food hygiene are very long and complicated.

*This doesn't say a lot for the state of the country's hygiene if long and complicated laws have to be passed to get results!*

The laws are open to a lot of interpretation and many people say that they have been designed to stop people opening food premises. This is perfectly true!

The people they have been designed to put off are those who are untrained, unqualified and are only interested in profit rather than running premises which are clean, hygienic and offer good wholesome food.

Of course if these people ran their premises in accordance with the health and hygiene laws and regulations their business would be that much more profitable and successful.

What do the various acts and regulations apply to?

◆ The production or sale of unsound, unfit or injurious food

◆ The prevention of contamination

◆ The hygiene of food premises, personnel and equipment

◆ Hygiene practices, including temperature control and heat treatment

◆ The control of food poisoning and food-borne disease

◆ The composition and labelling of foods

◆ The control of temperature is carried out for the storage of certain foodstuffs, particularly dairy and dairy related products

# Food Safety Act 1990

The Food Safety Act 1990 came into force on January 1st 1991. Some of the main points of this act are:

◆ That it is now an offence not only to sell unfit food but to have unfit food on food premises

◆ That Environmental Health Officers now have much greater powers to close dirty and unfit food premises

◆ That greater penalties can be imposed for offences against the *Food Safety Act 1990*.

*Local Environmental Health Officers* can apply to the courts for a **PROHIBITION ORDER** which allows them to shut down any food premises, within three days, which are not hygienic and pose a threat to public health.

# The Food Hygiene (General) Regulations 1970

The standards of food hygiene within food premises are controlled by these regulations, *but remember*, they are the basic, minimum standards and there is no reason why you should not always try and improve and advance these standards!

The main purpose of these regulations is to prevent the outbreak of food poisoning or food-borne disease and they are divided into the following areas:

FOOD HANDLERS

PRACTICES

PREMISES

EQUIPMENT

WASHING FACILITIES

SERVICES

PENALTIES

## FOOD HANDLERS

◆ Must be clean

Must cover cuts with coloured waterproof dressings

Must wear suitable protective clothing

Must not smoke or spit

Must report to superiors if they are suffering from food poisoning or a food-borne disease

◆ The superior must then inform the local *Environmental Health Officer*

## PRACTICES

These cover all restrictions on exposing food to risk through contamination *especially* keeping *high risk foods* under refrigeration and out of the danger zone and covering all open food offered for sale.

## PREMISES

Must be kept clean

◆ Must be kept in good repair

◆ Must be proofed against entry of food pests

## EQUIPMENT

◆ Must be made of non-absorbent materials

Must be maintained in good condition

◆ Must be kept clean (especially food containers)

## WASHING FACILITIES

Wash hand basin for personal use of food handlers must be provided in addition to sinks for washing food and equipment

These wash hand basins must be kept in a clean condition and provided with suitable soap, nail brush and drying system;

Hot and cold water or hot water at a controlled temperature must be provided at all sinks

## SERVICES

◆ A satisfactory supply of treated water must be provided

◆ Satisfactory first-aid materials must be provided

◆ Accommodation for outdoor clothing must be provided outside of the food area

◆ Sanitary conveniences must be well ventilated, lit and kept clean

◆ Sanitary conveniences must have hand washing facilities directly next to them

## PENALTIES

*All* offences are now punishable, on conviction with fines up to £20,000 *for each offence*. Sentences of up to 2 *years imprisonment* and unlimited fines can be imposed for serious offences.

*Now complete
the following questions at your own pace.
When you have completed the questions check your
answers by reading through Section 15 again.
Mark your answers using the
answer grid at the end
of package*

**I** Food premises can legally be closed if they

 *a* have no toilet facilities for customers
 *b* have no fridges
 *c* are very dirty
 *d* do not offer vegetarian foods

**2** Under the food laws which of the following *does not have to be provided* in food premises?

a first aid kit
b wash hand basin
c microwave oven
d separate area for outdoor clothing

**3** Which one of the following MUST be provided in food premises by law?

a shower facilities
b cooking facilities
c freezer facilities
d separate hand washing facilities

**4** Which one of the following could you be prosecuted for under the *Food Laws*?

a wearing dirty overalls
b smoking in the staff room
c causing an accident
d suffering from food poisoning

**5** Food premises must contain separate washing facilities for hands, equipment and food. TRUE/FALSE

# *Environmental Health Officers*

*Environmental Health Officers* are responsible for making sure that all food legislation is enforced. They are very highly qualified and experienced people and are always available to give advice and assistance to help you operate to high standards of food hygiene.

It is far better to ask for their help before outbreaks occur rather than call them in to investigate an outbreak of food poisoning or food-borne disease.

> **You should notice that under the *Food Hygiene (general) Regulations 1970*, all the statements use the word 'must' and not 'should' or 'could'.**

It is a legal requirement that these regulations are carried out!

*The penalty will be fines up to £20,000 for each offence and possible imprisonment.*

---

**Remember!! Your carelessness could cause an outbreak of food poisoning if you don't put into practice what you have learnt in this training package.**

---

Read through the whole training package again and concentrate on any section which you find more difficult than others.

The training package is there for you to use to make absolutely sure that you understand everything which you will need to know so that you can gain success in your examination, so do read it through as often as you need to.

*Knowing* how to carry out high standards of food hygiene and *actually* putting that knowledge into practice are two different things.

Always be alert for the opportunity of improving standards in your work place and passing on to others, the valuable information you have received.

It is only when *everyone* practices high standards of food hygiene that the increasing number of outbreaks of food poisoning and food-borne diseases will stop.

*Now complete the ENDTEST. When you have completed the ENDTEST, mark your answers using the answer grid at the end of the ENDTEST.*

*If you achieved a score of 19 or less then you need to go over the package again.*

## *ENDTEST*

You should arrange to complete the ENDTEST under as near examination conditions as possible – no distractions from television, stereos, other people etc.

Allow yourself a maximum of 40 minutes to complete the ENDTEST.

Answer *all* the questions by ticking one of the boxes against each question.

For example:

At what temperature do bacteria multiply most rapidly?

*a* 100°C
*b* 65°C
*c* 37°C
*d* 5°C

Take your time reading through each question carefully before selecting the answer.

GOOD LUCK!

**1** What temperature should the inside of a freezer be?

*a* 100°C
*b* 65°C
*c* 18°C
*d* −18°C

**2** What temperature should the inside of a fridge be?

*a* −18°C–5°C
*b* 1–4°C
*c* 50–60°C
*d* 30–37°C

**3**  Which of the following temperatures is within the '*danger zone*'?

 *a*   82°C
 *b*   37°C
 *c*    4°C
 *d*  − 18°C

**4**  When food is stored in a fridge, bacteria

 *a*  die
 *b*  multiply very slowly
 *c*  multiply very quickly
 *d*  do not grow at all

**5**  It is recommended that large pieces of meat are cut into smaller joints so that they

 *a*  carve more easily
 *b*  cool quickly
 *c*  do not shrink so much whilst cooking
 *d*  are easier to prepare

**6**  Food poisoning bacteria will multiply quickly in

 *a*  the fridge
 *b*  the freezer
 *c*  hot serving counter
 *d*  the kitchen

**7**  Fresh cream cakes should be handled with

 *a*  clean tongs
 *b*  clean hands
 *c*  wooden spatula
 *d*  palette knife

**8**  A food handler who has a cut finger must cover it with

 *a*  a clean bandage
 *b*  a finger stall
 *c*  a coloured dressing
 *d*  a coloured waterproof dressing

**9**  When should you wash your hands?

After you enter the kitchen (1)
After you dice some stewing steak (2)
After you prepare some sandwiches and then go for a break (3)
After you return from your break (4)

*a*  after 1, 2, 3
*b*  after 1, 2, 4
*c*  after 2, 3, 4
*d*  after 1, 3, 4

**10**  Washing your hands after smoking will help to prevent

*a*  salmonella bacteria
*b*  clostridium bacteria
*c*  staphylococcus bacteria
*d*  all these bacteria

**11**  A large piece of meat has just been removed from the oven, for use cold to-morrow. How soon will it be placed in the fridge?

*a*  within 24 hours
*b*  within 12 hours
*c*  within 3 hours
*d*  within $1\frac{1}{2}$ hours

**12**  Which of the following could do the job of a disinfectant?

*a*  detergent
*b*  sanitiser
*c*  iced water
*d*  water at 60°C

**13**  Bacteria need which one of the following to grow?

*a*  light
*b*  air
*c*  warmth
*d*  nitrogen

**14** Which of the following statements is true?

    *a* contaminated food looks and tastes normal
    *b* bacteria need light to multiply
    *c* all bacteria are harmful
    *d* all bacteria produce spores

**15** When can you return to work after suffering from food poisoning?

    *a* after 2 weeks
    *b* when you feel well enough
    *c* when you have been cleared by your doctor
    *d* once your course of medicine is finished

**16** Which one of the following foods would support bacterial growth?

    *a* uncooked rice
    *b* powdered milk
    *c* chutney
    *d* boiled ham

**17** When dealing with rubbish it is important to

    *a* keep the bins covered with a lid
    *b* store food waste separately
    *c* wash the bins daily
    *d* always use polythene liners in the bins

**18** Detergents are used for

    *a* completely removing all traces of bacteria
    *b* removing scratches on chopping boards
    *c* removing dirt, grease and debris
    *d* reducing bacteria to safe levels

**19** Which of the following are *common* symptoms of food poisoning?

    *a* fever and headaches
    *b* fever and nausea
    *c* stomach pains and headaches
    *d* diarrhoea and stomach pains

**20** How does food bacteria enter food premises?

a on pets
b on people
c on raw foods
d all of these ways

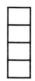

**21** The main reason why food pests should be controlled is

a they spread disease
b they make cleaning more difficult
c they cause food spoilage
d they are difficult to kill

**22** Most cases of food poisoning are caused by

a poisonous plants
b chemicals
c bacteria
d foreign objects in food

**23** Which one of the following materials should not be found in food premises?

a stainless steel
b copper
c formica
d wood

**24** Which one of the following helps towards kitchen hygiene?

a leave all spillages to dry before cleaning up
b use equipment as little as possible
c clean up as you go
d never use chemicals in the kitchen

**25** Which of the following are signs of a rodent problem?

a droppings, eggs, mould
b droppings, greasy marks around pipes, fur
c droppings, mould greasy marks around pipes
d droppings, eggs, greasy marks around pipes

**26** Food waste and refuse should be removed from food areas

a regularly throughout the day
b continually throughout the day
c after lunch and dinner service
d when staff are available to empty it

**27** Which one of the following MUST be provided in food premises by law?

a hot water at controlled temperature
b showers for staff
c rest room for staff
d stainless steel work benches

**28** For which one of the following could you be prosecuted under the food laws?

a having a cold
b smoking in the kitchen
c using cotton towels to dry your hands
d not reporting there are food pests on the premises

**29** Which of the following hand washing facilities must be provided in food premises by law?

a soap and hot and cold water
b soap, hot and cold water and a nail brush
c soap, nailbrush, drying facilities
d soap, hot water, nailbrush and drying facilities

**30** Food premises can now be closed down very quickly if they

a have no refrigeration facilities
b have no toilet facilities for customers
c are very dirty
d do not allow staff suitable break periods

# ENDTEST ANSWERS

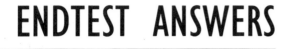

1 *d*, 2 *b*, 3 *b*, 4 *d*, 5 *b*, 6 *d*, 7 *a*, 8 *d*, 9 *b*, 10 *c*,
11 *d*, 12 *b*, 13 *c*, 14 *a*, 15 *c*, 16 *d*, 17 *a*, 18 *c*, 19 *d*,
20 *d*, 21 *a*, 22 *c*, 23 *d*, 24 *c*, 25 *b*, 26 *b*, 27 *a*, 28 *b*,
29 *d*, 30 *c*

# REVISION EXERCISE ANSWERS

### SECTION 1

1 Bacteria  2 Detergent  3 Disinfectant  4 Contamination
5 Cross-contamination  6 Food handler  7 Food poisoning
8 High risk foods  9 Sanitiser

### SECTION 2

1 *b*
2 *a*) Harmful, Cooking
  *b*) Contamination, Bacteria, Poisons
  *c*) Multiplication, Bacteria, Illness, Spoilage

## SECTION 3

1 *a*) WC, *b*) Raw, Cooked  *c*) Combing  *d*) Entering, Handling, Food  *e*) Smoking, Blowing  *f*) Refuse
2 True  3 True  4 *d*  5 *d*  6 *b*

## SECTION 4

1 *a*  2 *b*  3 *d*  4 *d*  5 Binary fission  6 *d*

## SECTION 4A

1 *a*) Onset time/Incubation period
  *b*) Duration of illness
  *c*) Symptoms
2 *c*  3 TRUE  4 TRUE  5 TRUE

## SECTION 4B

1 TRUE  2 *c*  3 TRUE  4 TRUE  5 TRUE  6 *b*  7 TRUE

## SECTION 4C

1 TRUE  2 FALSE  3 TRUE  4 TRUE  5 *b*  6 *b*

## SECTION 5

1 FALSE  2 *c*  3 *b*  4 FALSE  5 TRUE

## SECTION 6

1 *a*  2 *d*  3 *c*  4 *a*  5 *b*  5 *a*

## SECTION 7

1 *a*) The person  *b*) Raw foods  *c*) Insects  *d*) Rodents
  *e*) Animals  *f*) Birds  *g*) Dust  *h*) Waste food  *i*) Refuse
2 *b*  3 *b*  4 *a*  5 *c*  6 FALSE

## SECTION 8

1 *b*  2 *a*  3 FALSE  4 *c*  5 Stock rotation  6 FALSE
7 FALSE  8 TRUE  9 *b*  10 Raw meat and fish/cooked foods/ dairy products
11 *d*  12 FALSE  13 *a*  14 FALSE  15 FALSE  16 TRUE
17 TRUE  18 FALSE

## SECTION 9

1 *d*  2 *c*  3 *d*  4 *c*  5 FALSE  6 *d*  7 TRUE  8 *b*

**SECTION 10**
1 TRUE  2 TRUE  3 *d*  4 TRUE  6 TRUE  7 TRUE  8 TRUE

**SECTION 11**
1 TRUE  2 FALSE  3 *c*  4 *b*  5 *c*  6 TRUE

**SECTION 12**
1 *d*  2 TRUE  3 *b*  4 TRUE  5 FALSE  6 FALSE

**SECTION 13**
1 *c*  2 *b*  3 *c*  4 *a*  5 *d*  6 *c*  7 *b*

**SECTION 14**
1 *b*  2 *d*  3 *c*  4 *d*  5 *d*  6 *c*  7 Food and shelter

**SECTION 15**
1 *c*  4 *c*  3 *d*  5 *a*  5 TRUE

# FOOD HYGIENE – TEN GOLDEN RULES

 **ALWAYS** wash your hands before and after handling food, and always after using the toilet.

 **TELL** your boss at once of any skin, nose, throat or bowel trouble.

 **ENSURE** cuts and sores are covered with waterproof dressings.

 **KEEP** yourself clean and wear clean clothing.

 **DO NOT SMOKE** in a food room. It is illegal and dangerous. Never cough or sneeze over food.

 **CLEAN** as you go along. Keep all equipment and surfaces clean.

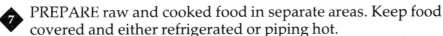 PREPARE raw and cooked food in separate areas. Keep food covered and either refrigerated or piping hot.

 **KEEP** your hands off food as far as possible.

 **ENSURE** waste food is disposed of properly. Keep the lid on the dustbin and wash your hands after putting waste in it.

**TELL** your supervisor if you cannot follow the rules. **DO NOT BREAK THE LAW**.

*The above text is reproduced by kind permission of Dept. Health and MAFF. It first appeared in the leaflet entitled, 'The Food Safety Act 1990 and You: A Guide for the Food Industry.'*